Prof. em. Prof. Dr. med. habil. Karl Hecht

Answers to
100 questions on
the healthy effect
of natural zeolite

SPURBUCHVERLAG

Answers to 100 questions on the healthy effect of natural zeolite

Prof. em. Prof. Dr. med. habil. Karl Hecht

Bibliographic information of the German National Library

The German National Library lists this publication in the German National Bibliography; detailed bibliographic data can be found on the internet http://dnb.dnb.de.

1st edition April 2016
© Spurbuchverlag, 96148 Baunach
info@spurbuch.de, www.spurbuch.de

Typeset: pth-mediaberatung GmbH, Würzburg
Cover design and layout: Monika Glück

ISBN 978-3-88778-479-9

You can find further books on the topics health and alternative medicine on the internet **www.spurbuch.de.**
Get our programme "Aktiv & Gesund leben" [Live actively & healthily] now – on the internet or via **info@spurbuch.de.**

Contents

Preface

The publication of the following books

- Hecht, K.; E. Hecht-Savoley (2005/2008): Naturmineralien, Regulation und Gesundheit. Schibri-Verlag, Berlin, Milow. 2nd edition, 424 pages, ISBN 3-937895-05-1
- Hecht, K.; E. Hecht-Savoley (2008): Klinoptilolith-Zeolith – Siliziummineralien und Gesundheit. Spurbuchverlag, Baunach; 2nd edition 2010, 3rd edition 2011
  ISBN 987-3-88778-322-8

has led to a growing interest in the silicates natural zeolite, bentonite/montmorillonite and silicon dioxide (synonym: silicic acid) on the part of therapists and especially on the part of the consumers owing to the healthy and quality-of-life improving effect of the silicates. According to various studies, the trend to orientate towards natural remedies leads to a growing demand of more and more people. However, the reorientation towards other remedies involves several questions. This also applies to natural zeolite, bentonite, montmorillonite and silicon dioxide (silicic acid), partly because of wrong ideas about the silicates that are often spread without any criticism and that cause insecurity among the people. Silicates belong to the oldest remedies of mankind e.g. in form of clay and medical clay. In fact, 2,400 years of experience have been gained already.

As the mechanisms of action and effects of such natural remedies are fundamentally different from those of traditional medical drugs, which are usually applied by conventional medicine, the need for knowledge is exceptionally great here. The number of requests that we have received almost daily over ten years proves that. This enormous interest has inspired us to answer the questions in written form and publish them as a book in order to satisfy the "thirst for knowledge" with regard to natural zeolite, bentonite/montmorillonite and silicon dioxide (silicic acid).

All the answers to questions from everyday life are, for the most part, put in easy terms for reasons of a better understanding. At the same time, however, they reflect the current scientific state of knowledge, which is documented in detail with all corresponding references in the book "K. Hecht: Lebenskraft durch das Urmineral Zeolith. Prävention, Detoxhygiene, Ökologie", published by Spurbuchverlag at the same time. You can read this comprehensive book in addition to deepen your knowledge.

During the 60 years of my career as a doctor and medical scientist I always followed the principle to recommend remedies and methods only after having tried them on myself. This also applies to natural zeolite and bentonite/montmorillonite. I have taken natural zeolite alone

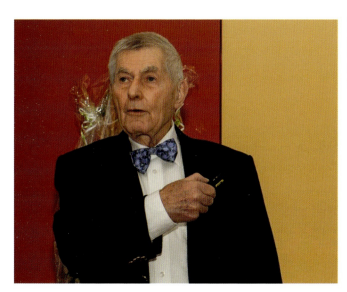

The author during a lecture at a colloquium on the occasion of his 90th birthday.

or combined with montmorillonite every day since the year 2000. At the age of 91 I can say that I am physically and mentally fit. Creative and sportive activities (such as Nordic walking) are part of my everyday life. Acquaintances of mine from different parts of the world who meet me after having not seen me for a long time use to say that I do not turn older but younger. In fact, this remark is confirmed by many results on the biological age. It has already been known in ancient times that silicates (clay minerals, bole) can have a "rejuvenating" effect. They are considered as the oldest most effective remedy and cosmetic of mankind.

The scientific findings of the American silicon researcher Edith Muriel Carlisle (1918-1996) prove that silicon dioxide molecules are part of the genes and that they stimulate growth and regeneration processes of human beings since the embryonic period. Silicon dioxide is actively involved in the protein synthesis of humans and animals.

In first place, the biological ageing process is caused and accelerated by a shortage of silicon dioxide. A shortage of silicon leads to a number of different diseases including – among other things – dementia, joint pain, osteoporosis, arteriosclerosis and skin diseases. Those, however, who take minerals containing silicon on a regular basis are able to balance this natural shortage, which is a normal consequence of the calendrical ageing process, and therefore remain younger and healthier in psychobiological terms. Furthermore, they can protect themselves against many chronic diseases.

Karl Hecht (*1924)

Important note

Medicine is a science that has always been subject to change-related developments for hundreds of years.

The information provided here on therapies and dosage recommendations, therapy models and forms of application are based on the most recent scientific state of knowledge and many years of experience on the part of the author and various therapists. Considering that medicine is an individual discipline and that according to practical experiences the same active agent can vary in its therapeutic effect depending on the individual, neither the author nor the publishing house can accept responsibility for the content. Therapists are advised to read all product descriptions and data sheets of the silicates natural zeolite and montmorillonite closely and to adapt the treatment to the individual. Those who are interested in natural silicates are advised to consult a therapist before taking them.

Acknowledgement

I am grateful to my wife Elena Hecht-Savoley for all her findings and ideas on this book resulting from many productive, critical conversations and the supportive role of her vision. I would like to thank her for that.

Also Dipl. Ing. Anke Dahmen has contributed in a well-known way to the success of this book. I am very thankful for the creative, technical design. I would like to thank my colleagues Dr. sc. med. Hans-Peter Scherf and Dr. med. Axel Kölling as well as my nephew, the natural healing practitioner, Peter Krönert for the precious input. I am particularly grateful to Gudrun and Juha Mermerci whose generous support enabled the English version of this book. I would also like to thank Klaus Hinkel for inspiring me to write this book and ensuring publication by the Spurbuchverlag.

Berlin, June 2015   Prof. em. Prof. Dr. med. habil. Karl Hecht

1_What inspired you to work on zeolites?

During my career as a doctor and scientist I have been inspired by some fundamental scientific findings and practical experiences:

- When I worked on research projects about the effects of psycho-pharmaceutical agents as a young doctor I realised that sooner or later I would come into conflict with the Hippocratic claim "Primum non nocere" (in English: do not harm as a doctor) by applying "chemicals" on sick people and accepting their side effects. This has motivated me to look for gentle natural remedies.
- Various research projects in the field of space medicine have made me aware of the significance of minerals for the fitness of human beings. I realised: minerals should be part of any therapy model. There is no life process without minerals. Minerals are the battery of human beings.
- Getting familiar with the outstanding research results of the American silicon expert Edith Muriel Carlisle and the Russian silicon expert H. G. Voronkov and his research team on the significance of silicon dioxide for the health of human beings.
- The successful application of zeolite and montmorillonite after the disastrous nuclear meltdown in Chernobyl (Ukraine). After the nuclear disaster in Chernobyl in 1986 500,000 tons of zeolite (which corresponds to a full freight train with a length of 124 km) were applied with the intention to decontaminate the released radionuclides. In addition, all people affected by the radiation disaster were also treated with zeolites, the sooner the treatment started, the better for the people. From that time on, I have been interested in zeolites and other aluminium silicates.

2_What are silicates?

First of all, silicates are very stable silicon-oxygen compounds that contain other very stable elements such as aluminium (which is the third most frequent element on our planet), magnesium, iron, sodium etc. The simplest silicate is silicon dioxide (SiO_2). SiO_2, which is also called silicic acid, has already been used very effectively in the human body. Other silicates that are important for human beings are natural zeolite and montmorillonite, also known under the terms bentonite and smectite. Owing to my experiences with their application as a preventive and therapeutic remedy I would like to compare their interaction to that of fraternal twins. When combined, they have a wide range of effects in the human body, whereas each twin contributes to the overall effect with a shared and individual characteristic.

However, there are more silicates than those that have been mentioned so far. More than 40 aluminium silicates are part of the very fertile soil of the earth's crust: clays, loam and loess.

3_What is natural clinoptilolite-zeolite?

Natural zeolites are natural microporous rocks of volcanic origin that can be found in certain mountains in many countries. Altogether, there are more than 100 different types of zeolites. The clinoptilolite-zeolite, hereafter referred to as natural zeolite, which is chiefly used for health-improving and medical reasons, belongs to the so-called crystalline forms. The basic skeleton of the clinoptilolite-zeolite is a crystal lattice with calibrated hollow spaces of about 4.0-7.2 Ångström (1 Ångström = 0.1 nm). The crystal lattice (part with the anions) consists of silicon (SiO_4) and aluminium (AlO_4) tetrahedrons. These solid SiO_4-AlO_4 crystal lattices that have a netlike shape consist of cations such as calcium, magnesium, sodium, potassium etc. and crystal water (not unbound H_2O). So far, at least 34 minerals have been detected in natural zeolites (clinoptilolite-zeolites), however, often in traces, which is exactly what a highly developed living organism needs.

4_What is montmorillonite/bentonite?

Bentonites are a white or grey white type of clay that is rich in minerals. The term derives from the place where they were discovered: Fort Benton, Montana, USA. Bentonites are so-called "sheet silicates" that originate from volcanic tuff containing silicon as a result of "weathering" and the impact of gravel bacteria, lichen and fungi, with montmorillonite as a main component. Montmorillonites were called after the place where they were supposedly discovered, the town Montmorillon (Vienne) in France. Pure montmorillonite has a grey white colour and is also characterised as a sheet silicate, just like bentonite, with anions from SiO_4 and aluminium (AlO_4) tetrahedrons. The ratio of silicon to aluminium in natural zeolites and montmorillonites is usually 3:1 to 8:1.

Montmorillonite, which originates from volcanic tuff, has outstanding effects for humans and animals.

5_What is the difference between bentonites and montmorillonites?

Normally, bentonites and montmorillonites (also called smectites) occur as a mixture of both silicates, however, at different percentages. There is a general international agreement on the terminology, i.e. all types of sheet clay with < 50 % montmorillonite have to be called bentonite. If the percentage of montmorillonite is > 50 % the term montmorillonite has to be used instead. A high percentage of montmorillonite is better for medical reasons because of its healing effect. The bentonite from Kazakhstan, which is certified in Germany and Russia, has a percentage of 95 % montmorillonite. For this reason, it has to be called montmorillonite. In order to test the quality of montmorillonite, montmorillonite powder has to be put into a glass of water. The quality is good when the powder starts to clump and is difficult to dissolve. Afterwards, the liquid has to be steered until the powder has dissolved. Now the liquid is ready to be drunk. As already mentioned, smectite is another term for montmorillonite.

6_How does the rough-structured zeolite become a consumption-friendly powder?

It takes three steps to produce a consumption-friendly powder. First of all, the zeolite rock is cut into smaller pieces and freed from foreign substances. Secondly, the natural zeolite is pulverized by means of micronization processes. Scientific examinations [Montinaro et al. 2013] and practical experiences with PMA zeolite show that an average grain size of approximately 7 μm is most effective in the human body. Thirdly, each charge is analysed and equipped with a data sheet. The data sheet reveals, among other things, the mineral and chemical composition, and confirms the absence of toxic substances and germs.

A zeolite grain consists of many tiny crystal lattice channels with a size of 0.4-0.72 nanometres. It looks like a sponge and can absorb ions like a sponge. The tiny channels are strictly calibrated and play an important role in the selective ion exchange. The selective ion exchange is not only important for the vital functions in the human body but also very interesting for technology. The production of synthesised zeolites according to the model of natural zeolites for a technical selective ion exchange has already become commonplace nowadays, the synthetically produced zeolites, however, are not suitable for human beings and should therefore not be applied here. (See question 87, p. 84 "Are synthetically produced zeolites interesting for health and medicine?").

The following picture shows a typical zeolite mine (Gördes, Western Turkey).

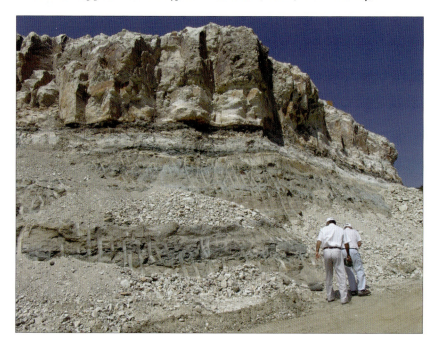

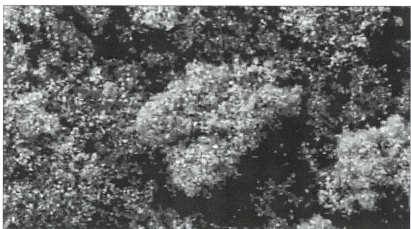

Natural clinoptilolite-zeolite grains with a diameter of approx. 10 μm in 300-fold magnification (modified according to Pavelič et al. 2004)

7_Scientists, doctors and the media claim that aluminium silicates are toxic and cause Alzheimer's disease?

These claims are based on the views of so-called fringe scientists who only deal with a certain aspect of a topic, while ignoring the big picture and the complex interrelations. As a consequence, they come up with wrong conclusions that sooner or later turn out to be wrong. My experiences with it are that the vast majority of people prefers to believe in such wrong ideas rather than the truth, and that such ideas persist for years despite all evidence that proves that they are wrong. The same applies to the hypothesis about the relation between aluminium and Alzheimer's disease.

Unfortunately, the times have not changed since Johann Wolfgang Goethe, our famous poet, as you can read in one of his famous wisdoms: "Truth must be repeated continuously, because error also is being preached all the time; and not just by the individual, by a large number of people. In the press and in encyclopaedias, in schools and universities – everywhere error holds sway! Feeling happy and comfortable – in the knowledge of having majority on its side." (Johann Wolfgang Goethe 1749-1832)

In case of aluminium silicates, this is the truth:
- They do not have a toxic effect for the human body.
- They do not have anything to do with the cause of Alzheimer's disease. On the contrary, they can even prevent it.

The scientific state of knowledge with regard to the aluminium silicates natural zeolite and montmorillonite briefly outlined.

As a matter of fact, aluminium silicates, e.g. in form of terra sigillata (medical clay), belong to the oldest and best practically proven remedies of mankind. They have been applied from the antiquity to the present without any documented undesired side effects during its application [Lange 2012].

In medicine, there is no other remedy than the aluminium silicates that has been applied practically and effectively, and tested for more than 2,400 years without any undesired side effects. Bentonite (Montmorillonite) has been applied for decades as a pharmaceutical remedy (adjuvant), detoxificant and sorbent in human medicine and veterinary medicine, especially in case of diseases of the digestive system. For this reason, also natural zeolite is added to medical drugs.

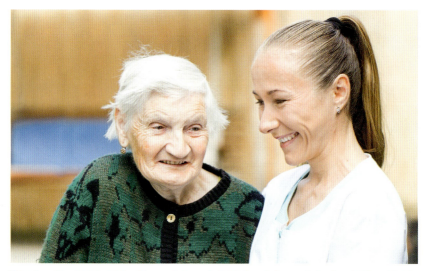

Natural zeolite, which is rich in silicon, protects against Alzheimer's disease. A shortage of silicon dioxide and intake of sleeping pills cause senile dementia.

In the last 20 years, the silicates natural zeolite and montmorillonite have been applied more and more often in more and more countries (such as the USA, Germany, Switzerland, Russia, Austria, Croatia, Italy, Spain, Monaco, Ukraine and Azerbaijan) with the intention to improve and maintain health, and as a basic therapy for the re-establishment of health and detoxification in a polluted environment.

In the USA, zeolites and aluminium silicates are permitted by the FDA (Food and Drug Administration), a federal agency of the United States Department of Health and Human Services. Zeolite registration number: 21(182.2727; aluminium silicate registration number: 21(182.2227. Apart from that, zeolites and aluminium silicates can also be found in the GRAS (Generally Recognized as Safe) list [Deitsch 2005].

Several scientists like White et al. [2008] from the famous Cambridge research group found out that aluminium ions have a strong affinity (attraction) towards the SiO_2 molecule with the result that they form very stable chemical compounds. What is more, silicon has a detoxifying effect with respect to aluminium. In general, it is not the amount of aluminium in aluminium silicates that plays a role but the ratio between silicon and aluminium. To put it in another way, if the ratio of silicon is higher than that of aluminium there is absolutely no danger of getting an aluminium intoxication. When zeolite and montmorillonite reach the human stomach the aluminium, which is released at a pH level of 4-6, is bound in the duodenum within a short period of time (6-10 minutes) at a pH level of > 8 as aluminate (e.g. antacids) or/and coupled firmly to the SiO_2 molecule. In zeolites and montmorillonites, Si and Al are organised like tetrahedrons (SiO_4 and AlO_4). During the release in the stomach, colloidal SiO_2 is formed (antacids = acid-binding agents, neutralisers). The US-American silicon researcher Edith Carlisle [1986] proved in experiments on rats that the toxic effect of aluminium can be totally eliminated and thus also the risk of a potential formation of plaque in the brain, which is often considered as a characteristic of Alzheimer's disease, but only on condition that there is sufficient silicon in the brain. Montinaro et al. [2013] proved in an animal experiment that oxidative stress leads to the formation of plaque in the brain and that this process, and thus also Alzheimer's, can be prevented with a permanent intake of natural zeolite, which is rich in silicon.

The French research group around Gillette-Guyonnet [2005] found out in an experiment with more than 7000 women older than 70 that the consumption of water that is rich in silicon improves the mental performance of older people and can prevent dementia. When low in silicon it increases the risk for dementia significantly. Drinking water containing silicon can remove accumulated aluminium from the human body.

8_You write that water containing silicon can remove aluminium from the body?

Yes, it can. The medical journalist Bert Ehgartner reports about it in the magazine Naturarzt [natural doctor] with the heading: Aluminium is an "alien" for the immune system.

Alien = extra-terrestrial being. He also writes about Al compounds in vaccines. In his interview Bert Ehgartner provides instructions, so to say, on how to protect oneself against an Al pollution and how to remove it from the body.

He comes to the following conclusion: "A removal of aluminium always makes sense. Up to present, there have only been a few relevant studies on the methods of removal. It is verified, however, that the consumption of mineral water that is rich in naturally dissolved silicon dioxide binds significant amounts of aluminium and removes them along with the urine. It cannot be confirmed, however, if aluminium can also be removed from sensitive organs like the brain, for example."

Bert Ehgartner is a strong supporter of Al toxicity. As the heading of his interviews already suggests, he portrays it as a demon.

9_Are aluminium silicates not having a high percentage of aluminium?

According to the scientific state of knowledge, not the absolute amount of aluminium is significant for the assessment of the biological effect of Al silicates but the ratio between silicon and aluminium. In case of natural zeolite and montmorillonite, the ratio is usually $Si:Al = 3:1$ to $8:1$. Normally, the percentage of silicon in natural zeolite and montmorillonite is 66-75 % and the percentage of aluminium 8-15 %. Due to the excess amount of silicon, aluminium silicates have a detoxifying effect in the organism of humans and animals, fight the Al there, are absolutely non-toxic and, above all, do not have any undesired side effects, on condition that the intake recommendations are always followed. In fact, this has already been proved by a larger research group in the field of human nutrition research in Cambridge under the direction of Prof. Ravin Jugdaohsingh.

Furthermore, both aluminium silicates, which have volcanic origins, have particular biological mechanisms of action in humans and animals.

This includes

- selective ion exchange,
- adsorption (binding of toxins),
- detoxification,
- silicon supply,
- mineral supply,
- catalyst effect as well as
- anti-bacterial, anti-viral, anti-mycotic and anti-inflammatory effects.

Al silicates have different bio-regulatory functions in the human body.

10_Natural zeolite rich in silicon, is it a possible means against aluminium strain?

Yes, it is. This question can be answered by the immunologist Dr. Erwin Walraph who ran an immunology laboratory in Neubrandenburg. Dr. Erwin Walraph sent me a written personal statement on the aluminium silicon problem in connection with natural zeolite, which I would like to quote in parts: **"Aluminium has different affinities to the organs"** (binding attractions). Due to the fact that it generates insoluble phosphates, this element is also called "bone seeker". Bones and muscles have comparable tissue levels. In case of daily workers, not exposed to it for professional reasons, the lungs have the highest level of aluminium, the level rises, as it is in the case of the central nervous system, with increasing age. Apart from that, Al is also stored in the liver, heart and spleen.

As far as I know, the only non-toxic aluminium is the aluminium silicate. This includes natural zeolites. Two scientific statements of the EFSA from the year 2013 confirm the safety of natural zeolite-clinoptilolites (E1g568 previously known as E568). The natural zeolite was classified according to its definition by the Regulation of the European Commission (2004) and the implementation of a new EU regulation (2013) as completely harmless with regard to the health of animals and humans.

In a clinical study (randomised, placebo-controlled, double-blind) at the Medical University of Graz, the aluminium level in the serum was determined with PMA zeolite at the beginning and also at the end of a 12-week supplementation phase. There were no significant differences between the zeolite supplemented group and the placebo group. Furthermore, two long-term observations were carried out on consumers who supplemented at least 5 g of PMA zeolite for at least 1 year or 3 years every day. Seven of the participants had already consumed this amount for a period of more than 15 years. No increased aluminium levels could be found in the blood and the urine.

Pre-clinical studies that were carried out by Prof. Pavelic at the University of Rijeka show that increased aluminium levels in the plasma, liver and the lungs, caused by an intoxication with aluminium chloride, could be reduced significantly by means of administering PMA zeolite. Compared to that, control groups who did not get a treatment had increased aluminium levels. Similar results with SiO_2 were documented by the US-American silicon researcher Edith M. Carlisle [1986].

11_Considering that aluminium silicates are part of the earth in form of clay, loam and loess, aluminium has to be part of natural food, too?

What happens to Al compounds, which are taken in with the food and drinking water, in the human body?

In nature: plants contain aluminium. The following list proves that:

"Food	Aluminium level in mg/kg
tea (dried products)	385
cocoa and chocolate	100
salads	28.5
legumes	22.5
grains	13.7
canned mushrooms	9.3
cabbages	9.0
sausage products	9.0
canned vegetables	7.6
canned fruit	3.6
fish and fish products	3.3
fruit	3.1
baby food	3.0
cheese	2.9
fresh mushrooms	2.7
pepper, cucumbers, tomatoes, melons	2.2
potatoes	2.1
meat	1.2"

examples of aluminium levels in food [Bundesverband der Lebensmittelchemiker(innen) im öffentlichen Dienst: Aluminium in Lebensmitteln] (quote)

Aluminium is a trace element. Trace elements are natural substances for the human body that can be involved in the physiological metabolism. Normally, the major part of Al compounds (10-50 mg/day) that is taken in with the food and drinking water can be removed by the human body. As a consequence, the urine can sometimes have a higher level of aluminium than the blood or the hair. This proves that Al compounds are usually removed from the body in a natural way.

The absorption of aluminium by the human body, i.e. in the digestive tract, depends on numerous factors:

- pH level (low pH level = acidic environment facilitates absorption. Therefore, you should not take medical drugs, vitamins, minerals etc. with fruit juices, wines and other acidic food or drinks.)

  There is no risk with regard to silicate intake (natural zeolite and montmorillonite). Dissolved natural zeolite has a pH level of 7.2-8.0, neutralises in the stomach and creates a slightly acidic environment.
- type of Al compound (There are probably more than 1,500 Al compounds)
- solubility of the Al compound
- dosage of the aluminium compounds

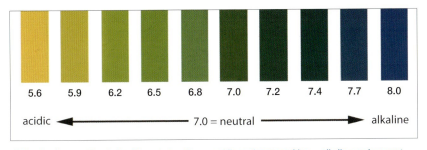

| 5.6 | 5.9 | 6.2 | 6.5 | 6.8 | 7.0 | 7.2 | 7.4 | 7.7 | 8.0 |

acidic ⟵――――――――― 7.0 = neutral ―――――――⟶ alkaline

pH level scale according to the litmus test. yellow = acidic environment, blue = alkaline environment

The Al compounds that are soluble and have entered the body are eliminated along with the urine [Thieme Chemistry 2013]. However, the Al compounds that are not soluble are eliminated along with the stool.

The EFSA and the BfR have the following opinion with regard to aluminium: according to the European Food Safety Authority (EFSA), the tolerated intake of aluminium per week is 1 mg per kilogramme body weight. A human being weighing 60 kilogrammes is allowed to

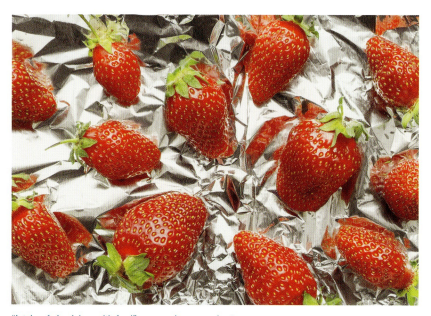

"Intake of aluminium with food": a normal process of nature.

consume 60 mg/week. Later, the tolerated level has been increased to 2 mg per kilogramme per week [EFSA 2013].

The amount of the consumed aluminium depends on the eating habits of humans. Under the designation E 173 aluminium is allowed as a food additive e.g. coats for sweets (sugar icing) and decoration of cakes. Also for colouring of medical drugs and cosmetics [Chemisches und Veterinäruntersuchungsamt Karlsruhe 2004; EFSA journal 2008].

Statement of the EFSA on the aluminium intake from food [2008]:

"Safety of aluminium intake from food. Scientific report on the part of the committee for food additives, flavouring agents, processing aids and materials that get into contact with food (AFC)." The EFSA journal (2008): 754, 3-4: "In fact, aluminium can be stored in different organs and in different tissues for a very long period of time until it is finally eliminated along with the urine…"

The EFSA and the Bundesinstitut für Risikobewertung [Federal Institute for Risk Assessment] assess the amount of aluminium that is taken in with the food every day as harmless, also with regard to Alzheimer's disease and carcinogenicity. The Food and

Drug Administration (FDA) of the USA declared aluminium silicates and zeolites in form of food supplements and food additives as harmless [Deitsch 2005].

Examinations in the laboratory indicate the following limit values:

blood	< 10.0 µg/l	(Labor 28 Berlin)
urine	< 22.3 µg/g	(Genova-Diagnostik)
hair	< 17.3 µg/g	(Genova-Diagnostik)

Of course, it can lead to an aluminium intoxication when these values are exceeded for a long time. This happens when technical aluminium is inhaled in production processes or as a consequence of a heavy overdose. The dose and the duration of exposure is an essential factor for toxicity (poisoning).

12_Aluminium is considered as a potential cause of Alzheimer's disease. Is that true?

The hypothesis about the relation between aluminium and Alzheimer's has been discussed controversially to its disadvantage for decades and neither accepted nor rejected as wrong by serious doctors, scientists, institutes and medical associations. The following quotes reflect the current medical-scientific state of knowledge:

Prof. Dr. Bauer: extract from his book "Die Alzheimer'sche Krankheit (Neurobiologie, Psychosomatik, Diagnostik und Therapie)"

Prof. Dr. Joachim Bauer is a specialist for internal medicine and psychiatry at the Psychiatric University Hospital Freiburg (Breisgau). Page 49, Alzheimer's disease, Schattauer Verlag, 1994:

"As far as toxins are engaged in Alzheimer's disease, the role has not yet been proven. All speculations about a pathogenic role of aluminium were mainly based on reports about higher morbidity rates in areas with a higher aluminium pollution of the drinking water [Martyn et al. 1986], on an assumed proof for aluminium found in plaques [Candy et al. 1986] and in neurofibrillary tangles [Good et al. 1992]. On the other hand, however, there were people who were heavily exposed to aluminium for different reasons without a higher risk of getting dementia [Rifat et al. 1990] and without a relation to neuropathology, which is a typical characteristic of Alzheimer's disease [Candy et al. 1992].

As it has been recently confirmed that plaques do not contain any aluminium and that previous measurements were based on contaminations of the examined tissue with fixatives containing aluminium [Chafi et al. 1991; Landsberg et al. 1992], a pathogenic role of aluminium is rather improbable."

The famous US-American Alzheimer's researcher Prof. Henry Wisniewski had the following opinion on the aluminium Alzheimer's disease hypothesis:
"There is no truth in it." "Every dollar that is invested in research is a lost dollar."

Henry Wisniewski died in September 1999. An obituary of Nick Ravo in the New York Times of 20/09/1999 contains the following words: "With his work he contributed a lot to fight the hypothesis that the use of aluminium at home or for the treatment of drinking water can cause Alzheimer's disease."

BfR [2005]
"No danger of getting Alzheimer's from aluminium in objects."

EFSA European Food Safety Authority
"Safety of aluminium intake from food. Scientific report of the committee for food additives, flavouring agents, processing aids and materials that get into contact with food (AFC)." The EFSA journal (2008): 754, 3-4:
"Based on present scientific data, diet-based exposure to aluminium cannot be seen as a risk factor for the development of Alzheimer's disease, according to the opinion of the committee…"

Alzheimer.de: information for patients and relatives
"It is a fact that many other factors do not contribute to the manifestation of Alzheimer's. This includes e.g. aluminium and other metals, infections, sexually transmitted diseases, hardening of the arteries, overload and underload."

Alzheimerforschung Initiative e.V.

28/07/2014

Risk factors for Alzheimer's disease:

- age
- genetics
- metabolic syndrome, cardiovascular factors
- diabetes mellitus type 2
- oxidative stress
- inflammations
- Aluminium is not mentioned.

Alzheimerforschung Initiative

06/03/2013

Dr. Mai Panchal, leader of the distribution of the funds at the AFI, says the following:

"A potential relation between aluminium and Alzheimer's is discussed very controversially in research. Tests with mice who were given aluminium did not lead to the manifestation of Alzheimer's disease."

"The research results of de Sole show, for the very first time, that ferritins of Alzheimer's patients have an increased aluminium level in contrast to the control patients. This does not say anything about the cause and effect. In the end, the increased aluminium level does not have to play a role in the development of Alzheimer's disease, but could be a potential consequence of it."

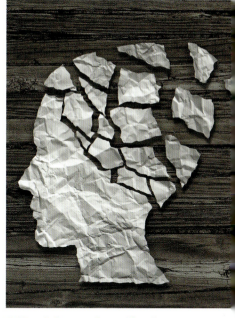

Alzheimer's disease = degeneration of the brain substance

"Ferritins bind themselves to many atoms and are a marker of iron deficiency in the blood. I do not think, however, that they are also a marker of Alzheimer's disease."

13_What could be the causes of senile dementia, occurring more and more often?

By integrating knowledge from conventional medicine, natural and alternative medicine, I would consider the following causes as being potentially involved:

1. Abuse of medical drugs, especially the intake of psychotropic drugs and sleeping pills (benzodiazepines).
2. Regular consumption of alcoholic drinks.

1. and 2. are often combined, which can lead to harmful interactions.
3. Gradual global intoxication with different environmental pollutants such as noise, electric smog and so on.
4. Lack of SiO_2, which is typical of old people, was proved by the French gerontologists under the direction of Sophie Gillette-Guyonnet [2005] as the cause of disorders of mental processes (degeneration).
5. Domination of oxidative stress and stress hormones subject to stress caused by psychological factors.
6. Insufficient use of the brain for creative activities (because of TV, internet) as well as lack of physical exercise [Manfred Spitzer: Digitale Demenz 2012].

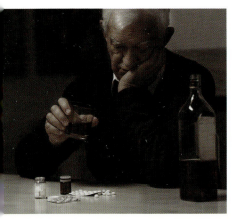 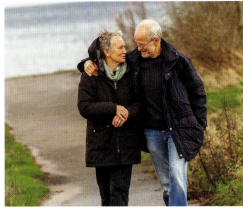

Potential cause of senile dementia: abuse of medical drugs and regular consumption of alcoholic drinks. Potential precaution: intake of SiO_2 and regular exercise in nature.

14_How can senile dementia be prevented?

Avoid medical drugs that increase the risk for dementia and luxury food, especially sleeping pills, psychotropic drugs and alcohol.

1. Take natural zeolite and/or montmorillonite, which are rich in SiO_2 and have a strong anti-oxidative and detoxifying effect, every day.
2. Be mentally active and creative.
3. Do regular exercise in nature.
4. Drink much water, especially water that is rich in SiO_2 (silicic acid).
5. Reduce the use of mobile phones to max. 20 minutes per day. Then switch them off! It has been proved recently that electric smog (radio waves) leads to oxidative and nitrosative stress [Warnke and Hensinger 2013; Yakymenko et al. 2014].

15_Could you explain ion exchange in a short and comprehensible way?

In general, ion exchange means that ionized (electrically charged) chemical elements are transformed from one medium to another e.g. from the body liquid serum to a tiny zeolite grain. Ion exchange is possible in one direction but can also be mutual. The mutuality of ion exchange takes place between zeolite grains and body liquids. Although ion exchange has already been described in the bible and even realised in technology for approximately 100 years it is still unknown to many people. For this reason, I would like to mention three interesting examples at this point.

Firstly: The second book of Moses says: "When they came to Marah; they could not drink the water of Marah because it was bitter. Therefore, it was named Marah. And the people grumbled against Moses saying: What shall we drink? And he cried to the Lord; and the Lord showed him a log; and he threw it into the water, and it became sweet." (Ex 15, 23-26)

How was that possible? By putting old (rotten) trees, which are good natural ion exchangers, into the water that contained magnesium sulphate (Epsom salt) in form of the natural mineral Epsom, the magnesium sulphate was removed with the result that the water lost its bitterness and became drinkable.

Secondly: The way Moses "sweetened" the bitter water with a piece of wood by removing magnesium sulphate, technology removes lead from the patrol with the help of synthetic zeolites according to the model of natural zeolite. If technology did not have the ion exchange of zeolites no car could drive with unleaded petrol.

Thirdly: Natural zeolite cannot only remove toxic substances from the human body in a selective way due to its tuff-based tiny channels (0.4-7.2 nm diameter), it can also nourish the minerals in the channels in a selective way. In general, ion exchange takes place on the basis of molecular and atomic bio-electrical processes. This is the first detox function of natural zeolite. Montmorillonite, however, leads to similar processes. In fact, both silicates ensure selective ion exchange. This means that only those ions (toxic substances) are removed from the human body that have to be removed and only those ions are provided that the human body actually needs.

16_Zeolite is associated with the sorbent function: what does that mean?

Adsorption is the second detox function of natural zeolite. Adsorbents (Sorbents) are capable of binding toxins and making them harmless. In medicine, "charcoal" has been used and is being used for this reason. With the help of charcoal I was able to help more than 30 people with a fungus intoxication to a better digestive tract during my student placement in 1948. Natural zeolite has a much stronger adsorption effect than charcoal and can make toxins, toxic substances, radionuclides and excess free radicals harmless. For this reason, zeolite also has an anti-oxidative function.

17_What are the most important functions of natural zeolite in the human body?

1. Selective ion exchange, which provides the amount of minerals that the human body needs for a systemic regulation. On the other hand, toxic substances are removed from the human body.
2. Adsorption, i.e. binding of substances e.g. toxins (poisons) that are made harmless. Both functions work together.
3. Colloidal silicon dioxide is provided.

18_What does colloidal mean?

As a general rule, the term colloidal stands for a particular condition of a liquid where the molecules are in a bio-electrical condition. In fact, all body liquids of human beings have a colloidal character: this includes blood, lymph, serum, tears, gall, gastric juices, urine and saliva. What is interesting, colloidal silicon dioxide from zeolites is adjusted to the respective body liquid. However, colloidal silicon has been identified as a controlling mineral of the connective tissue and therefore also called extracellular matrix.

Colloids can also have the form of gel. Joint cartilage, sinews and ligaments are gel colloids. This is why SiO_2 can be helpful in arthritis.

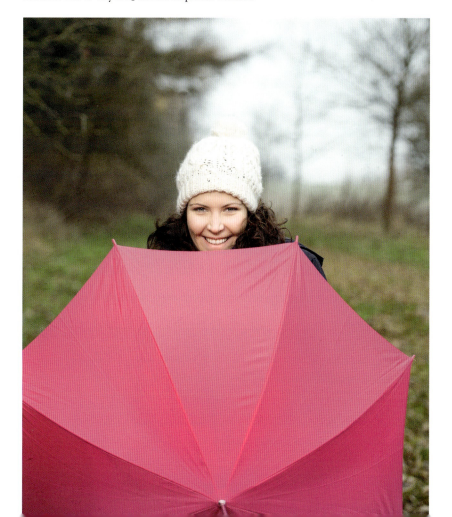

19_What is special about natural zeolites?

The micropores of tuff are equipped with tiny crystal lattice channels that have a diameter of 0.4-0.72 nanometres. They contain crystal water and anions of different minerals. The anti-oxidative effect is 160 times stronger than that of vitamin E. This can actually be proved with the help of the TEAC method (Trolox Equivalent Anti-oxidative Capacity). Natural zeolite can intervene in autoregulation of the human organism in a gently regulating way. This is a particular characteristic of the active agent.

The positive preventive and therapeutic effects of the clinoptilolite-zeolite, which have already been proved in several scientific papers, can be explained with the following six major functional characteristics:

1. Detoxification (removal of toxins) via ion exchange and adsorption
2. Necessary minerals are provided and the mineral metabolism is regulated
3. Electrolyte balance and bio-electrical activity via ion exchange
4. Removal of free radicals / anti-oxidative effect
5. Strengthening of the immune system
6. Colloidal SiO_2 is provided

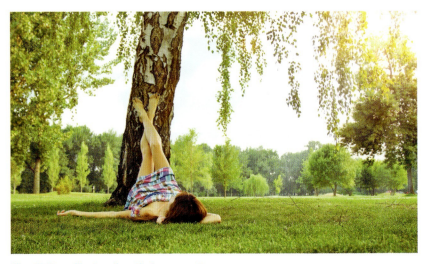

Clinoptilolite-zeolite strengthens the immune system.

20_Which functional characteristics of natural zeolite can be proved in the human body?

Natural zeolite:

- is good for detox hygiene
- controls and activates self-regulation and self-healing processes
- weakens undesired side effects of conventional medical drugs (chemotherapeutic agents, antibiotics)
- fights impotence and enables increase in libido
- binds heavy metals, ammonia, dioxin etc.
- activates the body's defence system
- improves the mental as well as physical performance and, apart from that, even performance endurance

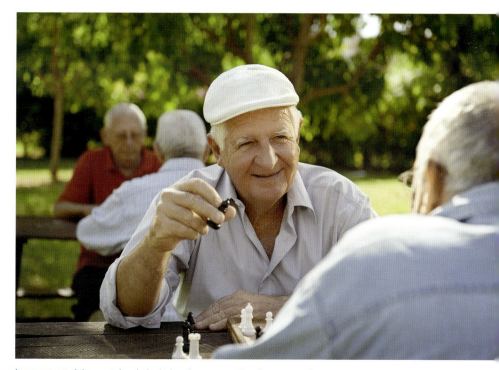

Improvement of the mental and physical performance, and performance endurance.

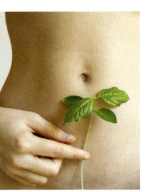 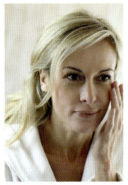 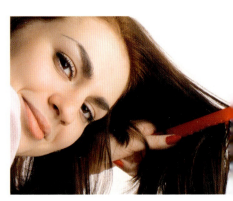

- is an active regulator of digestive functions
- protects against excess free radicals
- binds radionuclides of atom reactor rays
- ensures acid-base balance in the human body
- balances the electrolyte mineral metabolism
- can lift the skin and keep it young
- makes the hair glossy

In order to improve the effect of the silicate, a healthy lifestyle is recommended. In such a case, the effect can be improved.

21_What does healthy lifestyle mean?

- regular physical exercise (endurance sport)
- recreational sleep with a regular sleep-wake rhythm
- moderate diet that is appropriate for humans
- positive attitude towards life (optimism)
- stress management
- no luxury food
- no medical drug abuse
- sufficient nourishment with minerals, if possible, with silicates

22_What is actually the exact chemical composition of natural zeolites?

The chemical composition of natural zeolites can be different from mine to mine. The following table shows, for reasons of illustration, the exact chemical composition of the mine Nizny Hrabovec (Kosice, Slovakia):

Chemical composition			
SiO_2	65.0-71.3%	MgO	0.6-1.2%
Al_2O3	11.5-13.1%	Na_2O	0.2-1.3%
CaO	2.7-5.2%	TiO_2	0.1-0.3%
K_2O	2.2-3.4%	Fe_2O_3	0.7-1.9%

23_Can zeolite grains get into the cells?

As a matter of fact, no natural zeolite with an average grain size of 7.0 micrometres can get into the cells. The liquid in which the zeolite powder has been dissolved gradually passes the whole digestive tract from the oral cavity to the anus. The whole passage of the natural zeolite has been labelled isotopically and observed with adequate technology by Dr. Nikolai Daskaloff [2005]. During this passage in the digestive tract it comes to the selective ion exchange, the sorbent effect and the release of colloidal silicon dioxide via the intestinal mucosa into the connective tissue (which is also called extracellular matrix) and from there into the single cell groups. On the way back of the ion exchange, by-products, toxins and toxic substances are absorbed by the tiny zeolite grains. Finally, they are made harmless by means of adsorption and defecated.

24_How should natural zeolite be taken?

An ideal effect can only be achieved with the following method:
- Prepare a glass of water (warm).
- Put the correct amount of the powder into the water.
- Afterwards, stir the powder with a ceramic or plastic spoon long enough to achieve suspension.

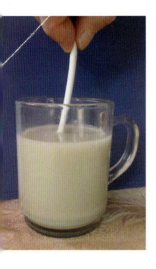

- Bring a small amount of the liquid (suspension) (approx. 20-25 ml) into your mouth. Keep it there for some time and then swallow it down slowly.
- Afterwards, stir the suspension again and bring a small amount of liquid into your mouth, keep it there for some time and then swallow it down slowly.

Repeat this process again and again until the glass is empty. Usually, one glass of water amounts to approximately 10-15 portions suspension, swallowed in sips.

Besides, you should drink 2-3 litres of water during the day.

stirring of zeolite powder to a suspension with a ceramic spoon

25_Which daily dosage is recommended?

The daily dosage for reasons of prevention can amount to 3 g for an adult. For people older than 50 6 g/day are recommended.

Experience shows that the daily dosage of 3 g should be taken directly after getting up, at least 1/2 hour before breakfast or before taking other active agents or consuming luxury food (coffee, tea, alcohol or cigarettes). In case of a daily dose of 6 g, half of the powder can be taken in the morning and the other half in the evening. The temporal distance to other substances (food etc.) should be at least 1/2 hour.

26_Can natural zeolite be drunk with fruit juice?

Please do not do that! Different fruit acids and enzymes, especially those of citrus fruits (grapefruit, orange, lemon, and mandarin) can influence the effect of the natural zeolite powder and lead to undesired effects. This recommendation does not only apply to natural zeolite or montmorillonite but to any active agent and especially medical drug.

27_Do natural zeolites have any side effects?

In general, no, they do not. They are absolutely non-toxic. Occasionally, however, they can lead to obstipations. This can be the case when insufficient water is drunk during the day. As long as enough water is drunk obstipation can be prevented. In such cases, a reduction of the dose should be taken into consideration.

28_Can natural zeolite be drunk with tea?

Natural zeolite can be drunk with green tea and herbal tea (warm), for example. Black tea and fruit tea are not recommended.

29_Can natural zeolite be also taken with other natural substances?

There is positive evidence for a combination of effects of natural zeolite and natural substances e.g. in case of:
- betanin (beetroot)
- spirulina alga (Spirulina platensis)

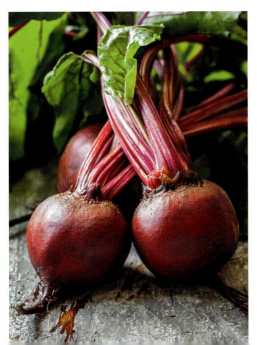
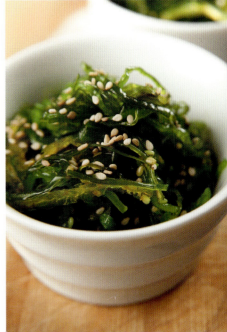

- microencapsulated glycine
- lycopene (substance of a boiled tomato)
- stinging nettle
- magnesium compounds
- bentonite/montmorillonite
- vitamin E
- chlorella alga

Furthermore, colloidal silicon dioxide from natural zeolite and vitamin C reinforce each other's biological effect.

30_Can natural zeolite be also taken with other medical drugs?

This has to be decided by the therapist and is different from individual to individual. Practical experiences show that natural zeolite can reduce undesired side effects of certain medical drugs. There is experience with natural zeolite in combination with antibiotics and chemotherapeutical agents. In fact, natural zeolite helped some cancer patients to avoid hair loss connected with chemotherapy. In any case, natural zeolite reduces or eliminates oxidative stress caused by medical drugs. Natural zeolite has a detoxifying effect and is gentle to

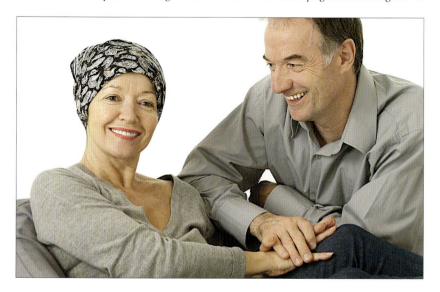

the liver when medical drugs are taken that are harmful to the liver. Ammonia, which plays a role in many disorders of the liver, can be adsorbed (bound). Also oxidative stress can be reduced or eliminated e.g. in case of diabetes mellitus. Patients with diabetes II were able to reduce their insulin dose or the dose of their anti-diabetic pills owing to the application of natural zeolite.

Natural zeolite, however, should be taken at least 1/2 hour before the application of any medical drugs.

31_Can natural zeolite be applied in patients with diabetes mellitus?

Also here, the therapist has to decide from case to case. Diabetes mellitus causes oxidative stress, which can be eliminated with natural zeolite. According to examinations, silicon dioxide, which can be found in natural zeolite and/or montmorillonite powder and enters the body in a colloidal form, can improve the function of the pancreas.

32_Can natural zeolite stop diarrhoea?

Also here, it is recommended to consult the therapist first. Practical experiences show that diarrhoea that is caused by wrong diets or food intolerances can be stopped with the application of natural zeolite. This can be achieved, for example, by taking 3-6 g of natural zeolite or montmorillonite in the described way. The best effect can be achieved with a mixture of both silicates 50:50.

33_Is natural zeolite able to trigger allergies?

No, according to the current state of the art and experience, it does not trigger allergies. Practical experiences show that natural zeolite can even prevent and eliminate allergies. For example, pollen allergies in spring, grass pollen allergies. The best anti-allergic results can be achieved with a combination of natural zeolite and spirulina platensis. Furthermore, there are examinations showing that natural zeolite powder can adsorb surplus histamine from the body and lead to an anti-allergic (against the allergy) reaction.

34_Can natural zeolite also eliminate enzymes, vitamins and hormones?

No! Natural zeolite and also montmorillonite can only remove smaller molecules from the body by means of ion exchange and adsorption. Hormones, vitamins and enzymes are characterised as large molecules. The selective (choosing) ion exchange is a particular and brilliant function of silicates.

35_For how many days/months can natural zeolite be taken?

As a general rule, it is recommended to take natural zeolite every day for 4 weeks. After this, a pause of 1 week should be kept. After the pause, natural zeolite can be taken for another 4 weeks. Further repetitions are possible. It is recommended to consult a therapist first. There are people who prefer taking zeolites for a short period of time because of the "sandy" taste. Personally, I have preferred a mixture of both silicates for more than 15 years every day, with the result that I feel comfortable with it.

36_Can natural zeolites affect the ability to drive?

According to the present state of knowledge, natural zeolites do not have any effect on the ability to drive. As they do not have a consciousness-impairing effect they can be taken in combination with driving a car. It has been proved in studies that natural zeolite can even stimulate the mental performance in a gentle way.

37_Can natural zeolite be taken with alcohol?

Alcoholic drinks should not be taken at the same time as natural zeolite. Natural zeolite powder can bind the alcohol in the body via ion exchange and adsorption, and thus make it harmless. There are study results that show that natural zeolite can be effective in case of alcohol intoxications. In such a case, higher doses are recommended. At least 6-12 g of natural zeolite per day for 4 weeks.

38_Is natural zeolite a universal remedy?

There is no such thing as a universal remedy: this is why neither natural zeolites nor mont-morillonites are universal remedies. Natural zeolite powder can have different effects in our body. For this reason, it is important to consider the individual needs of every human, as there is no "effect lumped together for all people". As a result, it is possible that natural zeolite works better for one person than for another. This is why it makes sense to look for the cause first. However, this should be done by the therapist. Sufficient water consumption and physical exercise can improve the effect of silicates.

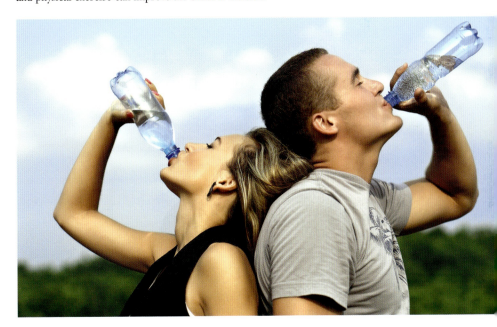

39_Can particles (tiny grains) of the natural zeolite powder get into the cells?

No. The tiny grains of natural zeolite are slightly larger than a μm. Nanoparticles are smaller than 400 nm. Such particles can get into the tissue and the cells. This is not the case in natural zeolite and montmorillonite powder.

40_What happens if higher doses of natural zeolite than recommended are taken?

The particular mechanisms of action of natural zeolite make sure that excess substance, i.e. the substance that is not needed, is simply defecated with the stool. An overdose with natural zeolite is impossible.

41_What are the different fields of application of natural zeolite?

The manual for zeolite science and technology [2003], written by Prof. Kresimir Pavelic and Dr. Mirko Hadzija (Croatia), mentions the following effects:
- anti-bacterial effect (against pathogenic bacteria)
- development and mineral development of the bones (bone health)
- neutralisation in case of excess gastric acid
- immune-modulating effects, strengthening of the immune defence
- reduction of the blood sugar level and anti-oxidative effect in case of diabetes mellitus
- blocking effects with regard to tumour growth
- binding of radionuclides (radioactive substances)
- Natural zeolite is non-toxic. It does not have any undesired effects that are harmful to the health of human beings.
- Furthermore, natural zeolite does not have any harmful effects on the embryo during a pregnancy.

42_Why is healthy longevity only possible with a non-toxic human body?

Above all, those who want to stay healthy and crave for healthy longevity, have to be free of toxins and metabolic by-products. An experiment of the French Nobel prize winner Prof. Dr. Alexis Carrel (1873-1944, Nobel Prize 1912) proves that healthy longevity is possible but only on condition that there are no "toxins" or, as he found out, no toxic metabolic by-products in our body.

Carrel kept embryonal chicken cells in a solution that contained all necessary natural substances. In order to eliminate the metabolic by-products, he exchanged the solution

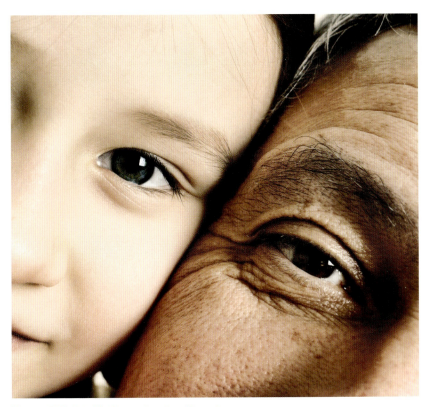

Young and old: detoxification can slow down the ageing process.

every day. While chicken normally live approx. 7 years, these chicken cells lived 29 years. Most probably, they would have lived longer, if one of Alexis Carrel's assistants had not forgotten to renew the solution every day. **This was the fundamental experiment of detox hygiene.**

On the basis of his interesting observations, Dr. Carrel drew the conclusion that the ageing process can be prevented or at least slowed down by removing all the harmful by-products (in form of a detoxification). According to Carrel's point of view, the ageing process is caused by an accumulation of toxic substances in the human organism. Later, the findings of Dr. A. Carrel were repeatedly confirmed by other doctors. This is why detox hygiene is an essential part of a healthy lifestyle and juvenile ageing.

43_What basic conditions are the typical indications of an intoxicated human body?

First of all, toxins cause inflammations e.g. as a basis for cancer diseases. Furthermore, they also cause oxidative stress, i.e. excess unbound O_2 and NO (nitrogen monoxide) radicals that, in such a form, can be very aggressive with respect to the cells and the genetic structure of the human body.

Apart from oxidative stress and nitrosative stress (excess nitrogen monoxide radicals, NO), also environmental pollution causes the so-called dismineralosis. The term dismineralosis stands for a disturbed mineral balance that can cause different kinds of chronic diseases. Furthermore, dismineralosis is caused by the toxins that remove important minerals from the human body. When minerals, for example magnesium, are taken, they are removed from the body for the most part due to dismineralosis [Ziskoven 1997]. For this reason, one should always follow the principle "Detoxification should precede a diagnosis". As soon as the toxin has been removed from the human body, which has to be confirmed by means of specific tests, of course, a clean diagnosis can be made. For this reason, detox hygiene is very important and should always be part of a healthy lifestyle.

44_What do free radicals do in the human body when they are present?

Accelerated breathing, degenerative diseases of the nervous system, blocking of spermatogenesis (formation of sperm cells), arteriosclerosis, mitochondrial diseases, increased susceptibility to virus infections, different types of cell damage, autoimmune diseases, skin disorders, eczemas, melanomas, diseases of the respiratory tract, malfunctions of the immune system.

45_What is detox hygiene?

Hygiene means maintenance of health, staying healthy, contributing to the maintenance of health. Detox hygiene, on the other hand, means maintenance of health by means of detoxification.

Hygiene was introduced by medicine with the intention to resist harmful germs that cause various diseases (in first place, this meant regular washing hands). Later, hygiene also embraced fighting (avoiding) all organic as well as non-organic pathogens. To put it into other words, this includes toxins that can be found everywhere: for the most part in the air, in the water and in the food.

The main target of hygiene is prevention for reasons of maintaining or even improving the well-being and performance of the human body. Detox hygiene accentuates this target with regard to the continually increasing gradual poisoning (intoxication).

46_What should be considered with regard to detox hygiene?

The detoxification system of the human body should be kept fully functional from an integral point of view. The detoxification systems of the human body are the liver, intestines, lungs, skin, kidneys, blood circulation and lymphatic system.

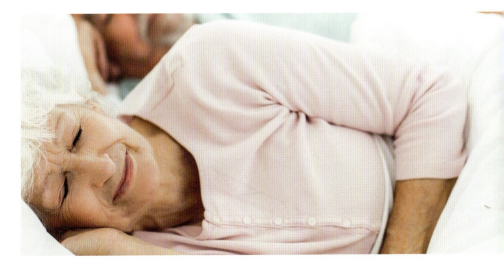

restorative sleep

According to WHO (World Health Organization) recommendations, a healthy lifestyle inclu-ding a correct and moderate diet, regular physical exercise (especially endurance sport) and restorative sleep while respecting, at the same time, a regular sleep-wake rhythm and avoiding so-called auto-intoxications (excessive tobacco use, consumption of alcoholic drinks and medical drugs) can make a big difference. Many people do not know that too many medical drugs can intoxicate a human being, too.

Detox hygiene also means:
1. Being aware of gradual intoxication.
2. Avoiding and fighting exogenous, toxic factors that can be influenced by the lifestyle, for example intoxication due to distress as a result of psychosocial, noise and electric smog stress factors.
3. Avoiding mass prescriptions of medical drugs. 1-3 medical drugs is the maximum a human body, especially an older human body, can tolerate.
4. Applying (taking) natural substances corresponding to the nature of human beings, are non-toxic, capable of detoxifying the tissue and the cells in an integral way and that provide all the necessary minerals at perfect doses. **Today, this can only be said of natural clinoptilolite-zeolite and montmorillonite as well as other silicates e.g. clay minerals.**

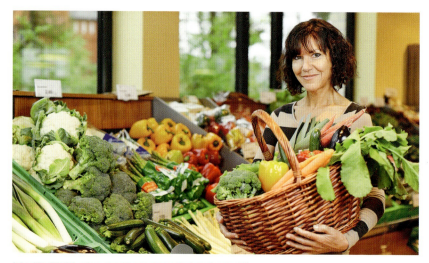

A healthy lifestyle also comprises a correct and moderate diet.

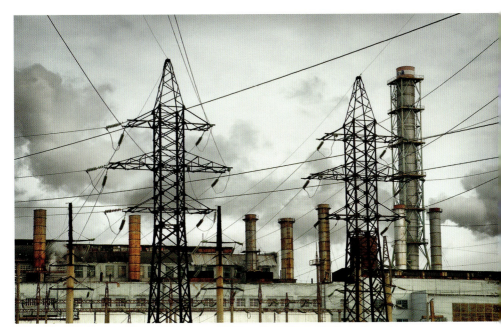

Toxic factors such as distress as a result of electric smog have to be avoided.

47_Why detox hygiene with natural zeolite and/or montmorillonite?

Detoxification of the tissue and the cells by providing minerals can be ensured with these two silicates in an ideal way.

Why is this necessary?

At the moment, there are factors causing global health problems:

1. **gradual intoxication**
2. **shortage of minerals in the food**

ad 1: The people currently living on our planet are exposed to gradual intoxication caused by different environmental pollutant. The toxic substances taken with the air by breathing, by drinking water and with nutrition.

Traces of toxins in food and drinks: drinks from plastic bottles contain bisphenols that can cause hormonal disorders, especially with regard to children. Men are in danger of

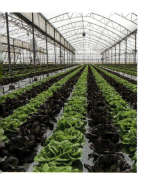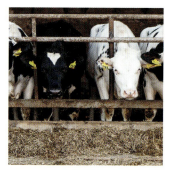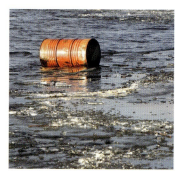

Over-cultivation of vegetables, livestock breeding that is not species-appropriate, environmental pollutants: loss of health, shortage of minerals and gradual intoxication in humans.

"feminising" due to the bisphenols, and get sexual disorders. Our food, drinking water and drinks contain different toxic substances, as can be learned from reports of different consumer organisations constantly published. This includes, among other things: preservatives, colouring agents, stabilisers, flavour enhancers, herbicides, and heavy metals e.g. lead in leaf vegetables.

The air contains soot particles with different chemical compositions of exhaust gases from vehicles and industry.

Home, furniture, carpets, paint and floors are also part of the human's environment. Often they contain toxic substances that are breathed in in traces by the humans every day. Furniture from plastic contains toxins (poisonous substances). New apartments often contain the toxic formaldehyde.

Noise, electro smog and radioactivity are totally underestimated by most people. They can reinforce the negative effects of the toxins in the human organism (lead to interactions). More and more celebrities are aware of gradual intoxication and protect themselves against it with the help of natural zeolite.

ad 2: Nowadays, most food offered in supermarkets does not contain the amount of minerals that it had 100 years ago because of over-cultivation of vegetables and fruit as a result of plant processing, unnatural soil cultivation and livestock breeding that is not appropriate to the species. The consequence is a dangerous shortage of minerals in humans and thus also loss of health.

48_What is gradual intoxication?

Gradual intoxication and a shortage of elementary vital minerals cause chronic diseases: allergies, autoimmune diseases, psychological disorders, neuro-generative diseases, and early biological ageing.

Furthermore, both health disturbing global influences cause oxidative stress (excess free radicals), which is another pathogenic factor that accelerates the ageing process.

In the famous anti-cancer book of the French physician

David Servan-Schreiber, researching in the USA, a whole chapter "Cancer and environment" is dedicated to the significance of environmental chemicals that play a role in the manifestation of cancer diseases. One of his most important therapy recommendations is: detoxification of the body of the person affected. It is much better to protect oneself with silicates and detox hygiene.

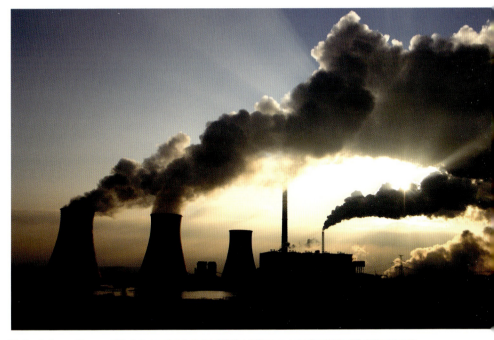

Toxic substances from coal-fired power plants make sick. The follow-up costs for the health industry and the economy amount up to 6.4 billion EURO in Germany every year (Deutsches Ärzteblatt, 03/05/2013, Volume 110, No. 18).

49_Are there studies on gradual intoxication?

Yes, there are. Here are some examples.

1. **Scientific results of a detox campaign of the European Section of the WWF**
[Campagne Detox of the WWF; World Wildlife Fund, 2005, www.panda.org/detox]. In the course of this campaign, the blood and urine of adults were examined on a large scale and voluntary basis with regard to 109 environmental chemicals. David Servan-Schreiber points out a person with 42 of 109 substances. I would like to quote another report of David Servan-Schreiber.

   "In the course of the study, 39 members of the European Parliament and 14 ministers for health and environment from different European countries were examined. Everybody, without exception, was contaminated with considerable amounts of toxic substances that are harmful for humans. 13 chemical residue products (phthalates and perfluour compounds) were found in all Members of Parliament, the ministers had traces of 25 chemical substances, among other things, flame retardants, two pesticides and 22 PCB (polychlorinated bisphenols). This type of gradual intoxication cannot be reduced to the representatives or Europeans: in the USA, scientists of the Center for Disease Control found 148 toxic chemicals in the blood and urine of Americans of all ages."
   Herbicides "sprayed" in fruit gardens

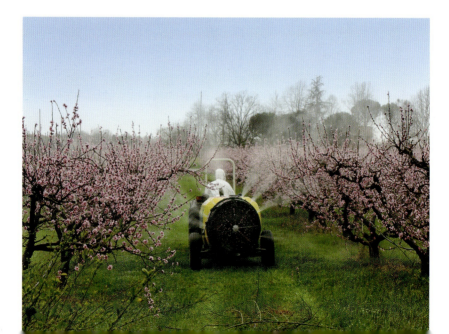

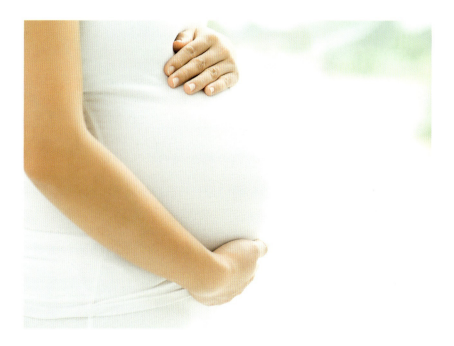

Toxins in the womb

The magazine Spiegel No. 39 of 27/09/2010 wrote: "Toxins in the womb!". This article reports about the US-American physician Frederica Perera who found out that environmental chemicals can enter the womb of pregnant women and cause damage to the foetus. The result is sick children.

This article from the Spiegel from the year 2010 also mentions results of a group of experts engaged by the US government. Blood and urine from adults were taken and analysed with regard to the presence of environmental chemicals. According to the report in the Spiegel, up to 212 chemicals were found in a few humans.

50_Are there studies proving that toxic substances are adsorbed (bound) by natural zeolite and thus decontaminated (made harmless)?

Serial examinations with pupils in a paediatric clinic in Chelyabinsk (Russia) proved that 16 % of the examined pupils had high and very high levels of Cd, Cu, Cr, Ni and Pb. A daily four-week application of natural clinoptilolite-zeolite freed the organism of the children from excess toxic substances successfully. This was confirmed by two follow-up examinations that were carried out after the application [Shakov 1999].

According to a screening examination, 102 of 157 (65.6 %) men were burdened with heavy metals. They received clinoptilolite-zeolite for 30 days, 2 x 1.25 g.

The results revealed that the cadmium, lead, copper, chromium and nickel levels in the blood were below the allowed limits after a 30-day treatment with natural zeolite. The author [Shakov 1999] concluded that not only the toxic substances were removed with clinoptilolite-zeolite, the self-regulation with regard to the optimisation of the homeostasis of the mineral metabolism of the whole organism was re-established.

Miners had increased concentrations of lead in the blood. For this reason, they were given 5 grams of clinoptilolite-zeolite for 25 days every day. The amazing result can be seen in the bar chart below.

The analysis of the lead level in the blood was carried out with the help of mass spectrometry with inductively coupled plasma. This is a very sensitive measuring method.

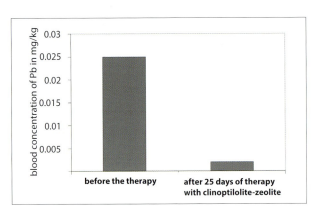

lead levels in case of miners before and after the therapy with natural zeolite [Veretenina et al. 2003]

Application of natural zeolite in case of alcohol intoxications: 50 of altogether 100 male patients with an alcohol intoxication who were treated with a common complex therapy obtained 2×5 g of natural clinoptilolite-zeolite every day in addition to the conventional therapy. During a 10-day therapy, the blood serum liver values GGT = gamma glutamyl transferase, ALAT = alanine aminotransferase and the ASAT = aspartate aminotransferase were checked on the 4th, 7th and 10th day of treatment. According to the results, the increased liver values, which are a normal consequence of any alcohol intoxication, normalised faster thanks to the addition of natural clinoptilolite-zeolite than the liver values of the patients who did not take this mineral. To sum it up, the therapy with zeolite was more effective and faster [Blagitko and Yashina 2000].

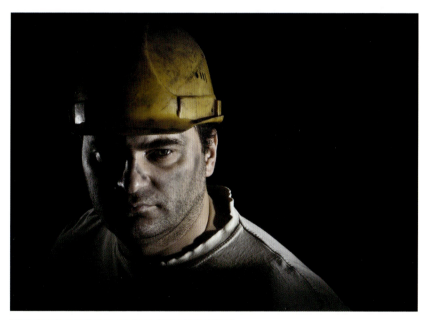

Miners had increased concentrations of lead in their blood.

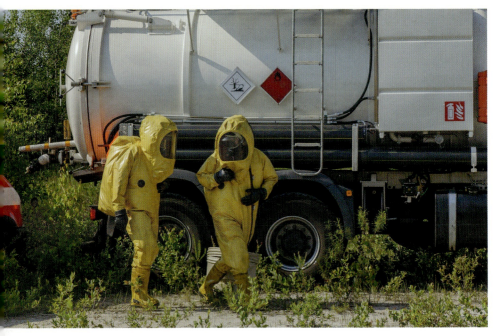

Contamination due to toxic substances

51_Are different toxic substances and toxins adsorbed (bound) by natural zeolites and also synthetic zeolites?

The field of zeolite application for the removal of toxic substances and toxins from the environment of the human and from the human body is extensive. The following list shows examples of relevant research results on adsorption via zeolites.

The following list, which is not intended to be exhaustive, stresses the versatility of natural and synthetic zeolites with regard to adsorption:

- arsenic
- mycotoxins
- alcohol intoxications
- worm eggs
- medical drug substances, side effects
- bisphenols (e.g. plastic bottles)
- toxic sulphur compounds

- methyl alcohol
- nitrogenous toxins
- radionuclides

Furthermore, there are reports on the elimination of toxic substances (lead, cadmium and caesium) from contaminated waste water systems with natural zeolite and synthetic zeolite in big cities. (Detailed references in the book: K. Hecht: Lebenskraft durch das Urgestein Zeolith. Prävention, Detoxhygiene, Ökologie. Spurbuchverlag.)

52_What are toxic substances?

In terms of everyday language, all substances that can have harmful effects for human beings, animals, plants and ecosystems, are referred as toxic substances. This definition, however, is fuzzy, considering that some substances or their effect can influence human beings in a positive way, on condition that certain circumstances are given, but also in a negative way when the circumstances are different.

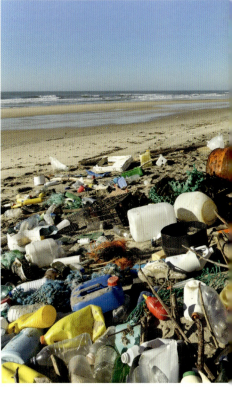

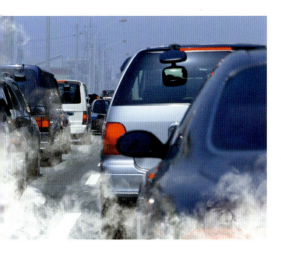

A famous physician from the middle ages, Paracelsus (1493-1511), postulated: it is the dose that makes the poison. But also the duration of exposure to toxic substances and toxins of human beings plays a decisive role. A one-time, short-term exposure to the substance can even have a positive effect on the human being. Constant exposure, on the other hand, can make you sick.

53_What are heavy metals? Are they always toxic (poisonous)?

Heavy metals are:

antimony	arsenic	lead
cadmium	cobalt	iron
gold	copper	manganese
nickel	plutonium	mercury
uranium	zinc	

Depending on the dose and the duration of exposure, heavy metals can cause intoxications in the human body. There are different classifications of the elements that belong to heavy metals. Some organisations or authors categorise lead, cadmium, mercury, arsenic, copper, nickel and manganese as heavy metals.

Some heavy metals are toxic in small doses (poisonous) e.g. arsenic, lead, mercury, antimony, others only in high doses. Heavy metals, however, are also classified as essential (necessary for the human being) trace elements, considering that they are absolutely necessary for the vital processes of humans in tiny amounts (traces) e.g. zinc, iron, manganese, lead and even arsenic.

This is why literature often refers to the fact that heavy metals are not principally or generally toxic, but as already mentioned, depend on the dose and the duration of exposure. The International Union of Pure and Applied Chemistry IUPAC [Duffus 2002] recommends to avoid the term "heavy metals", also the term "toxic substances" should not be used to replace it, as some of them are essential (absolutely necessary) for the health of human beings.

For this reason, there are set limit values for blood examinations that allow tiny amounts of heavy metals in the human body. If, however, the limits are exceeded, there is a higher risk of getting a heavy metal intoxication. **At the same time, it should not be the aim to achieve zero values with regard to heavy metals in the blood or in the human body. Nevertheless, it should always be kept in mind that heavy metal intoxications are very serious diseases.**

54_Could you provide some examples for limit values?

aluminium < 10.0 µg/l	nickel < 2.8 µg/l	vanadium < 1.1 µg/l
antimony < 7.00 µg/l	selenium 53-105 µg/l	zinc 60-120 µg/l
arsenic < 2.2 µg/l	silver < 0.3 µg/l	tin < 2.0 µg/l
lead	silicon > 190 µg/l	lithium 0.5-1.2 µg/l
men and women < 45 years < 10.0 µg/dl women > 45 < 40 µg/dl	strontium 10.0-70.0 µg/l	non-organic phosphate 0.8-1.45 mmol/l
		sodium 132-145 mmol/l
cadmium < 0.4 µg/l		potassium 3.5-5.1 mmol/l
chromium < 0.4 µg/l		calcium 2.1-2.6 mmol/l
cobalt 0.5-3.9 µg/l		chloride 96-110 mmol/l
copper 85-155 µg/dl		
magnesium 1.6-2.5 mg/dl		
manganese < 3.2 µg/l		
molybdenum 0.3-1.2 µg/l		
iron 33-193 µg/dl		

examples for limit values of elements in the blood of human beings

In order to prove toxic substances in the human body, the blood (present state), hair (chronic state) and the urine (elimination capacity of absorbed environmental pollutants) have to be examined with regard to the respective levels. In the best case, the human body is capable of removing a certain amount of the toxic substances that are taken in every day, especially when they are soluble. As a general rule, it is advantageous when a urine test reveals a high elimination capacity. As a consequence, it is disadvantageous when the levels in the blood and hair are high.

55_How was natural zeolite applied after the reactor disaster in Chernobyl?

Altogether, 500,000 tons of natural zeolite and a huge amount of montmorillonite were applied in Chernobyl after the reactor disaster. The water of the river Dnieper (in close proximity to Chernobyl) was freed of radionuclides (caesium 137) with natural zeolite. Also the drinking water pipelines were freed of radionuclides with natural zeolite within one year. Around the reactor, barriers were constructed that consisted of zeolite material with the intention to prevent contamination of the river in case of a flood. First, the soil in the area of the reactor was removed and washed, afterwards the washing solution was treated with the help of a special zeolite filter system. Vegetables were only cultivated in greenhouses where zeolite was added to the soil, with the result that the concentration of caesium 137 and strontium 90 in the plants fell by unbelievable 50-70 %.

Zeolite powder was also added to the animal feed (1-3 g of natural zeolite per kilogramme body weight). As a consequence, the concentration of radionuclides in the meat fell by 50-70 %, in the milk by 80-85 %. Zeolites in food for humans reinforced the removal of caesium 137 in the human body by the factor 3-5.

The Bulgarian scientist Ludmilla Filizowa reports on the 4th International Conference Natural Zeolite 93 in Sofia that she was able to reduce caesium 137 by 30 % by means of adding 10 % clinoptilolite-zeolite to cow's milk and decontaminate children of caesium 137 by means of adding 30 % clinoptilolite-zeolite powder to chocolate and cookies. Special washing machines were applied to wash clothes with a suspension containing zeolite [according to Malsy and Döbli 2004]. Apart from natural zeolite also the layered clay montmorillonite was used. Clothes, equipment, walls, roofs etc. were sprayed and washed of radioactive material with the help of suspensions made of montmorillonite.

Russian and Ukrainian scientists came to the conclusion that the main problem was that natural zeolite was not available from the beginning, because it had to be transported over thousands of kilometres. They found out that the effect of natural zeolite on people contaminated with radionuclides was better the sooner the application of natural zeolite started. They recommended to take natural zeolite on a permanent basis in order to protect oneself against radionuclides. I have done this myself for 15 years.

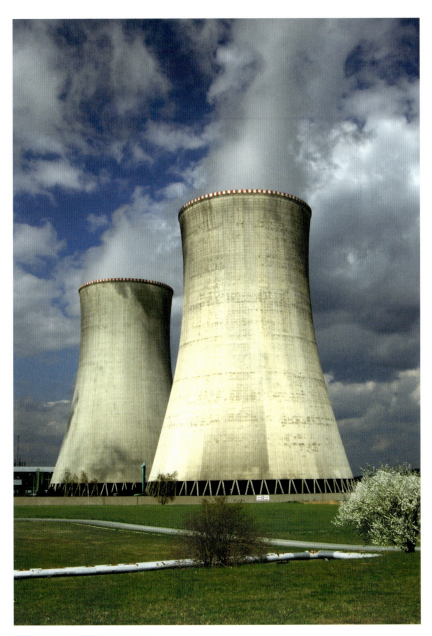

Radioactivity from nuclear reactors

56_Should all NPPs have zeolite reservoirs?

The findings from the nuclear disaster in Chernobyl should be used to oblige by law all NPPs that are currently in use to have reservoirs with huge amounts of natural zeolite in close proximity to the reactor for the case of emergency. Furthermore, the emergency reservoirs of natural zeolite should be stored separately and accessibly according to the following main focuses by all NPPs.

1. To extinguish the exploded block of the NPP.
2. To fight the emission of radioactivity from the reactor block that is damaged directly and successfully.
3. To prevent radioactive materials from entering the soil and water.
4. To wash all houses, vehicles, equipment, machines, clothes, livestock and other things that get into contact with radioactivity.
5. To protect contaminated food and drinking water that did not get into contact with radioactive material.
6. To protect livestock against radioactive contamination.
7. To prevent or treat symptoms of radiation in humans and animals.

57_Zeolite mountains for the final storage of nuclear waste?

On the basis of the experiences that were gained in Chernobyl with 500,000 tons of zeolite, it would make sense to consider this silicate in its tuff form as a temporary storage or final storage place.

There has been such a project in the USA for more than 10 years: the nuclear waste final storage Yucca Mountain in the State of Nevada. The Yucca Mountain is a mountain range with a length of approx. 10 km, consisting of more than 50 % clinoptilolite-zeolite. Experts who knew the decontaminating power of natural zeolite, suggested to store the US-American nuclear waste in Yucca Mountain as a final storage. In 2002, the US Senate under the presidency of George Bush decided to extend Yucca Mountain as a geological nuclear waste final storage. A tunnel was introduced into the mountain that is 200-400 m below the surface of the mountain and 150 m above the groundwater level.

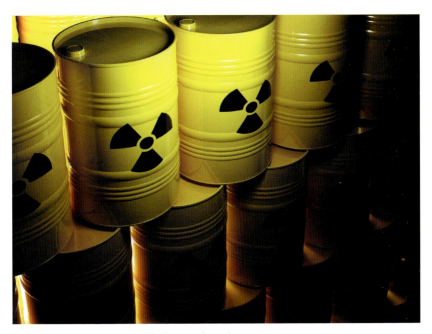

Zeolite as a temporary storage and final storage for nuclear waste.

The idea was to store 77,000 tons of radioactive nuclear waste and 63,000 tons of spent fuel elements there. Environmental organisations and inhabitants of the State of Nevada have fought against this project since the beginning of construction. The main argument: the area around the Yucca Mountain is not safe with regard to earthquakes and volcanic eruptions. In February 2009, president Obama stopped the project for the time being.

In my opinion, zeolite mountains are the safest final storage for nuclear waste, as they are not only storage places, but decontaminate radionuclides at the same time, i.e. can make them harmless. Of course, they have to be safe in case of earthquakes or volcanic eruptions.

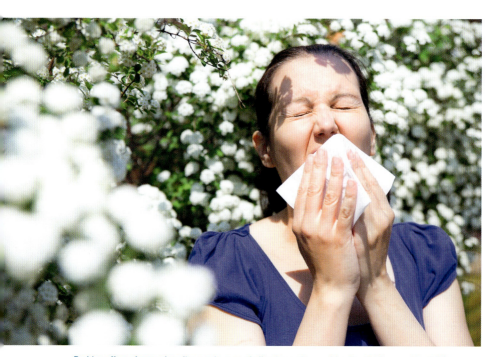

Positive effect of natural zeolite e.g. in case of allergies and wound healing (picture on the right).

58_Are there studies on the effect of natural zeolite in case of diseases?

Yes, there are many studies. The following list shows some of the positive effects of natural zeolite with regard to different diseases from the book of Prof. Dr. EM Blagitko and Prof. Dr. F. T. Yanshina, from the Russian Ecological Academy and the Novosibirsk Medical Academy with the title "Prophylactic and medical effects of natural zeolite" [2000] including information on the correct dosage.

- **For diseases of the immune system:** 70 kg body weight, for 7-8 days, 2-3 g daily; pause after one week: repetition of this application.
- **As a health care measure in case of pregnant women:** 1-5 g daily for 3 days; repetition of this application after one month.
- **For coronary artery diseases:** 5 g daily, for 3 days; 1 week pause. Then repetition of this application 3-4 times.

- **Hepatitis** (inflammation of the liver) (all types): 1.2-2.0 g every 2-3 hours for 3-4 days.
- **Allergies:** 0.5-1 g daily for 7-8 days. Afterwards, one week pause and repetition of the procedure.
- **Elimination of radioactive iodine in case of children:** 3 g zeolite every day for the duration of 18 days.
- **Healing of wounds after operations:** 1.5 g daily, for 3-14 days (depending on the need).
- **In case of bone fractures of the legs:** 3 g daily, for 6-7 days.
- **Skin diseases:** 2-3 g per day, for 5-12 days. Then one week pause and repetition of the application.

The zeolite powder was stirred to a suspension in a glass of water and drunk in sips (see question 24). This dosage recommendations originate from the beginning years of application of natural zeolite in medicine (2000). This is the reason why low doses were used. Later, higher doses were used.

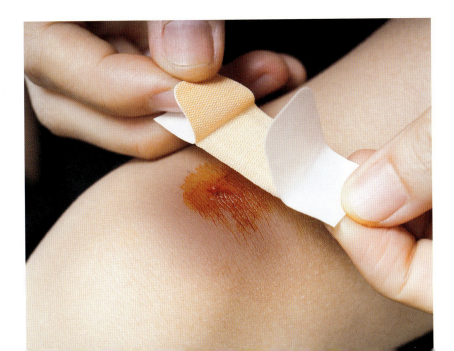

59_Are there studies on the application of natural zeolite and montmorillonite in case of diseases?

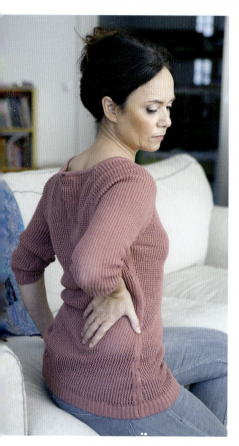

Application of natural zeolite in case of inflammatory diseases such as rheumatism.

Yes, there are many! There is a number of studies that proves the effective application in case of disorders and diseases of the digestive system. In case of diarrhoea, reflux (belching) and heartburn, both remedies worked effectively. Also montmorillonite was broadly applied in the field of veterinary medicine on pets with intestinal disorders.

Apart from that, there are also numerous studies on the effective treatment of the skin. In such cases, the silicates are applied internally and externally. This means that the silicates are taken with a glass of water and applied on the affected areas in form of suspensions (similar to solutions) or pastes. In fact, many dermatologists have come to the conclusion that skin diseases are caused by disorders or diseases of the intestines.

Since natural zeolite and montmorillonite have the capability to bind free radicals (which is also called oxidative stress), these silicates are applied for diseases where oxidative stress plays a role e.g. diabetes mellitus (sugar disease), inflammatory diseases and rheumatism.

The silicon, which is part of the silicates, leads to a good bone mineral density. For this reason, the application of natural zeolite has proved in case of osteoporosis.

60_Are there observations on the effects of natural zeolite in case of fungal infections?

The effect of SiO_2 in different fungal diseases has been known for many years now. Renata Bourbeck, natural healing practitioner in 83253 Rimsting, who carries out anti-fungal treatments according to Prof. Dr. Enderlein and, in addition, applies natural minerals, tested the effect of the natural clinoptilolite-zeolite recipes "Sanofit He" and "RelaxSan He" on patients with fungal infections with the help of a blood dark field microscope according to K. Hecht.

The effect of natural zeolite montmorillonite remedy recipe "Relaxsan" (according to K. Hecht) in case of a candida infection of the intestines

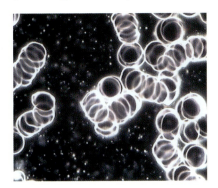 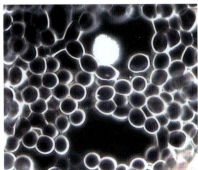

Before   After with Relax Scan

left: typical "intestinal roll of coins" of the candida and mucor racemosus fungi on the haemogram before the treatment.

right: after application of dissolved "RelaxSan" the "rolls of coins" were dissolved and the acids in the blood were neutralised.

Similar results were achieved with other natural zeolite recipes.

61_Is it possible to carry out a treatment with natural clinoptilolite-zeolite on patients with a smoker's leg and diabetic's leg?

Blagitko and Volkova [1999] report about the application of natural clinoptilolite-zeolite for the treatment of ulcers of the lower extremities (smoker's leg) of more than 50 patients. Also Čuikova und Voskakov [1999] achieved similar results with the application of natural zeolite in 20 patients with a so-called "diabetic's leg".

Here are two documented cases.

1. A Swiss "healer" called me one day and asked me for advice. He had a patient (forester by profession) whose "diabetic's leg" was planned to be amputated. The patient, however, refused to let the amputation be carried out. So I recommended to apply 10 g of natural zeolite every day instead, to observe the patient for 2-3 weeks and then decide whether an amputation might be necessary. Since I did not get a call 4 weeks after my recommendation, I called the healer. I asked him about the patient and he answered that he was back in the forest, doing his job. His leg was healed.

2. An 88-year old man had suffered from an "open leg" (ulcus cruris) for approx. 20 years. He went to the Turkish health resort NaturMed as a patient. We ordered daily baths in the thermal water that is rich in SiO_2 and a daily intake of 5 g of natural zeolite (mixture of zeolite and montmorillonite). After only 10 days the open wounds were healed. When the patient presented himself one year later, his leg was free of ulcus cruris wounds.

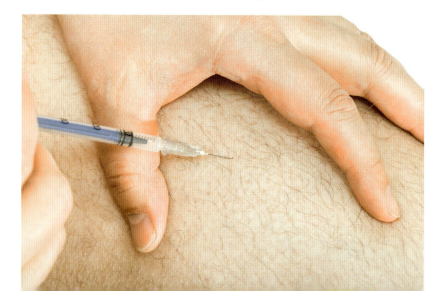

62_Has natural zeolite been applied on patients with tumour diseases?

There are many studies proving the healing effect of natural zeolite in patients with tumour diseases. Here are some examples:

Case controlled study renal cancer

[Ivkovic 2006]

- 23 cancer patients interrupted the therapy suggested by conventional medicine at the terminal stage despite two or more metastases at the bones, the second kidney, the lung and the brain.
- Constant therapy with natural zeolite
- Period: 8 years
- 3 patients died after 14 days of therapy.
- In case of 9 patients, the metastases shrank.
- In case of 8 patients, there was a total remission after 2 years.
- In case of 3 patients, the growth of the metastases was stopped.

A comparison to the group that was not given natural zeolite reveals that all patients died after one year.

Case controlled study prostate gland cancer

[Ivkovic 2006]

24 patients with primary prostate gland carcinoma: constant therapy with natural zeolite

Result

- All patients had lower PSA values after 2 months of therapy.
- In case of 7 patients, no tumour cells of the adeno carcinoma could be found in a biopsy after 2 months.
- 8 patients with metastases in the bones had:
  - improvement of the general state.
  - in case of 5 patients, there was a stopped growth of the metastases in the bones after 6 months.
  - in case of 2 patients, there were no metastases found after 6 months.
  - In case of 2 patients, no effect.

Dr. Ilse Triebnig (Villach/Carinthia) has treated more than 1000 cancer patients successfully with PMA zeolite within the last 12 years. The results are well-documented.

63_Can drinking water, containing SiO_2, prevent from tumour diseases?

It is a common fact that mineral sources or drinking water sources that contain silicon can prevent cancer diseases. F. Goldstein [1932] reported that Daun in Western Germany, where a mineral source contains 80 mg/l silicon dioxide, has a very low mortality rate with regard to cancer in contrast to other places in Germany. Voronkov et. al. [1975] report that the areas, where the drinking water contains little silicon, have a higher morbidity rate with regard to tumour diseases in contrast to places where the people were provided with water that contains natural silicon.

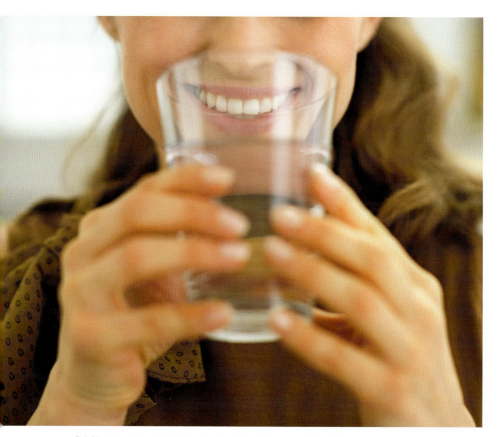

Drinking water sources or mineral sources containing silicon prevent cancer.

64_Why is silicon also referred to as being the original base mineral of our planet?

Following oxygen, silicon (as silicate and silicon dioxide) is the second most common element on our planet. The earth's crust most probably consists of 75 % silicates and 12 % silicic acid (SiO_2). Altogether, 800 different silicon compounds have been found. Among other things, quartz, rock crystal, amethyst, smoky quartz, morion, citrine, rose quartz, diatomaceous earth, basalt, mica, feldspar, opal, olivine belong to the silicic acid compounds SiO_2. Elementary silicon (Si) is very rare on our planet.

65_Which characteristics make silicon dioxide (also called silicic acid) so unique?

Silicon (SiO_4 and SiO_2) has versatile unique effects in the human body, which makes it significant advantageously different from other minerals in a positive way. The aluminium silicates natural zeolite and montmorillonite provide SiO_2 for the human being and lead to the desired effects. This includes the following:

- SiO_2 (silicon) molecules have a crystalline structure. The crystalline structure of SiO_2 molecules ensures, in functional (cybernetic) terms, an open system that all living organisms have in common. This way it can ensure biological functions without any difficulties or side effects.
- In fact, SiO_2 minerals have played a decisive role in the formation of all prototypes of life on earth.
- Silicon molecules can be found in the genes and are able to carry out different gene transactions.
- The crystalline structure of SiO_2 can radiate vibrations with different frequencies and achieve a natural bio resonance (see question 99).
- SiO_2 has a specific water chemistry. It is said to be capable of binding up to 40 times its weight to water. This is why firm skin, similar to the one of young people, can be guaranteed. Shortage of silicon leads to "wrinkling" of the skin with advanced age, as the specific water chemistry is reduced because of a shortage of SiO_2.

66_The Nobel prize winner Iljin Metschnikov (1845-1916) postulated: "You are as old as your connective tissue." Is there a connection with SiO_2?

Yes, SiO_2 is indeed the regulating mineral of the connective tissue. The age of the connective tissue is mainly induced by SiO_2 (silicic acid mineral) e.g. firm skin, glossy hair and smooth nails.

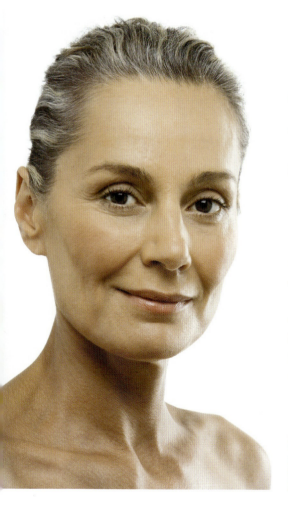

Due to the adsorption (binding) of proteins by the SiO_2 molecule and the involvement of the body SiO_2 in protein synthesis (protein growth synthesis), the SiO_2 can stimulate tissue renewal. The US-American silicon researcher Edith Muriel Carlisle [1986] was able to prove that. Furthermore, she discovered that silicon plays a decisive role in embryogenesis (development of the embryo), especially in growth. Edith Muriel Carlisle postulated: "There is no growth without silicon".

Also the specific water chemistry of silicon, which has already been mentioned, plays a role here. It has been proved scientifically: silicon is capable of slowing down the biological ageing process and preventing arteriosclerosis, wrinkling of the skin and calcification of the blood vessels. For this reason, silicon is also called "rejuvenating salt".

SiO_2 is the regulating mineral of the connective tissue and can stimulate tissue renewal, therefore it can slow down the biological ageing process.

67_The level of silicon in the body decreases with advancing age. Is there any proof for that?

Scientific literature provides the following quantitative indications on age-related presence of SiO_2 in the human body.

Baby: the highest concentration of silicon can be found in the umbilical cord. The skin, the connective tissue and all organs of the baby have high concentrations of silicon, leading to a firm netting of the connective tissue.

Adult: adults have high concentrations of silicon in the connective tissue, in the nails, in the lymph glands, in the eye lenses, in the hair, in the enamel, in the lungs, in the skin, in the bones and in the cartilages. The smooth muscles have more silicon than the cross-striped muscles.

Old person: old people have a shortage of silicon, depending on the biological age. It results, among other things, in wrinkling of the skin, less elasticity in the connective tissue, dull and dead hair, and brittle finger nails. These appearances are caused by drying of cell proteins, leading to a falling cell pressure [Voronkov et al. 1975; Scholl and Letters 1959; Carlisle 1986].

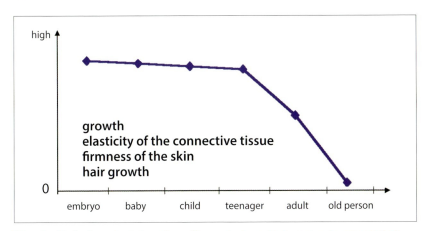

Silicon level in the human body depending on the age (semi-quantitative, schematic representation) based on literature research [Hecht and Hecht-Savoley 2005]

68_Are there studies on the retardation of the ageing process due to SiO_2 or the silicates natural zeolite and montmorillonite?

We reviewed the following questions in a random check:

1. Is it true that aged persons have a lower silicon level in the blood?
2. Will a long-term intake of clinoptilolite-zeolite and/or montmorillonite guarantee a constantly high silicon level in the blood?

First, we assembled a group of subjects who had taken silicates for a long time already, then, a control group, at similar age, i.e. elder people, who had never taken silicates to compare.

Altogether, 12 people, 4 females and 7 males, at the age of 48-90 were examined. They had taken doses of more than 5 g of one or both silicates on a permanent basis every day for 2-13 years. A female person, however, had to be excluded from the study, as she did not fulfil all the requirements. The major part of the 12 people (9 women, 3 men) who had never taken any silicates and thus served as the control group came from a residential area in Berlin (70 % retired people).

Since it was our general intention to find test persons who fulfilled certain criteria such as locomotor mobility (walking), mental activity, flexibility as well as self-care abilities for both groups, we knew that this task would become more difficult with regard to the control group, especially with regard to the men in the control group, as it is generally more difficult to find men that fulfil such criteria than women. Considering that a lot of men of that age did not meet the requirements as expected, at least in this residential area, there were mostly women in the control group. One reason could be the shortage of SiO_2, which is typical of older men.

The test persons 1, 2, 5, 6, 8, 11 and 12 had taken both silicates. The test persons 2, 7, 9 and 10 had only taken natural zeolite on a regular basis.

All 23 test persons had to give blood from the cubical vein on an empty stomach on two successive days (between 8 a.m. and 9 a.m.) in the laboratory "Labor 28", Mecklenburgische Straße 28, 14197 Berlin.

The analyses of the silicon in the blood were carried out with the help of atom absorption spectrometry. This is a very sensitive analysis method. The reference value of the laboratory was determined with > 190 µg/l.

The results are presented and assessed in the following table.

TP No.	1	2	3	5	6	7	8	9	10	11	12
Sex	F	F	F	M	M	M	M	M	M	M	F
Age	79	72	46	90	89	65	59	48	48	73	73
Duration of zeolite intake in years	>11	>6	>2	>6	>13	>3	>2	>2	>2	>2	>2
Silicon ref. value > 190 µg/l	451	580	509	576	596	362	354	362	374	503	500

TP No.	1	2	3	4	5	6	7	8	9	10	11	12
Sex	M	M	F	F	M	F	F	F	F	F	F	F
Age	69	72	76	76	82	73	62	57	76	61	50	56
Element												
Silicon ref. value > 190 µg/l	187	300	147	113	310	116	245	207	348	129	404	191

Silicon level in the blood in case of a long-term application of natural zeolite and montmorillonite.
Above: silicate group, below: control group (without silicates).

average value silicon **with** silicates   470 µg/l (> 70 years (N=6): 534 µg/l)
average value silicon **without** silicates   225 µg/l (> 70 years (N=6): 222 µg/l)

As can be derived from the table, a long-term and regular intake of the silicates clinopti-lolite-zeolite and montmorillonite can result in higher Si levels in the blood in contrast to people who do not take such minerals at all. The average value in case of the verum group was 470 µg/l. In case of the people older than 70, the average blood level of the silicon amounted to 534 µg/l (n=6).

Due to other present data one can conclude that the health state of the silicate group is better than that of the control group. (Detailed information in Hecht et al. 2014 in the magazine Orthomolekulare Medizin und Ernährung No. 148).

69_What are the conclusions?

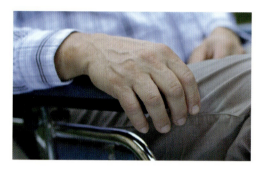

Examinations that were carried out with two groups confirm that older people who have a high level of silicon in the blood – in contrast to people with a lower Si level – have a better state of health.

1. Our random sample results confirm,
   - that the silicon level in the blood falls drastically with advanced age,
   - that a permanent intake of silicates in case of older people can help to keep the silicon level high and
   - that this high silicon level in the blood can result in a good state of health in older people.
2. Silicates (SiO_2, silicic acid, clinoptilolite-zeolite and montmorillonite) can serve as donators (suppliers) of the essential trace element silicon in a regulative way and compensate the age-relating loss of the endogenous silicon.
3. We would like to adjust the chart below due to the random sample results, as shown in the chart on p. 69.

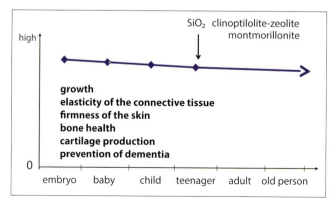

On condition that silicates are taken regularly on a permanent basis, the silicon level in the blood in case of older people can be maintained at the level of adults with the result that the biological ageing process is decelerated.

70_Could you present the oldest test persons of the above-mentioned silicon study? Yes.

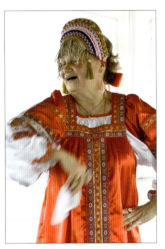 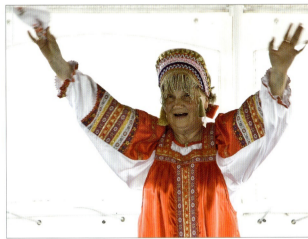

(pictures above) Elena, test person 1: after 11 years of daily intake of clinoptilolite-zeolite. 75th birthday: Kalinka dance

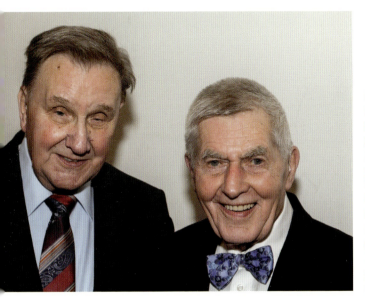

(F.l.t.r.)
Harry, Test Person No. 5:
91 years after > 7 years of daily intake of natural zeolite, thick hair, smooth skin, mentally fit, quick-witted, humorous.
His laboratory results are normal. He goes hiking for 1-2 hours every day.
Author, Test Person No. 6:
14 years daily intake of both silicates, natural zeolite and montmorillonite.

71_How do you know that your biological age is younger than the calendrical age?

- **Visual age = optical age**
  Smooth skin, face with a few wrinkles, body shape, posture
- **Biological ageing results**
  Bone mineral density, laboratory values, sleeping profiles, ECG, anti-oxidant capacity, silicon level in the blood etc.
- **Mental-emotional age**
  Memory, creativity, felt age, optimism, social communication
- **Activity age**
  Activity characteristics during walking, running, soft elastic walk
- **Speaking age**
  Loud, clear, light voice, fluent speech

72_Which groups of people have a particularly high need for SiO_2?

- pregnant women
- high requirements in job
- sportspeople, especially competitive sports
- permanently stressed people
- mal nourished people
- chronically ill people
- people with an infect tendency
  electro-sensitive people

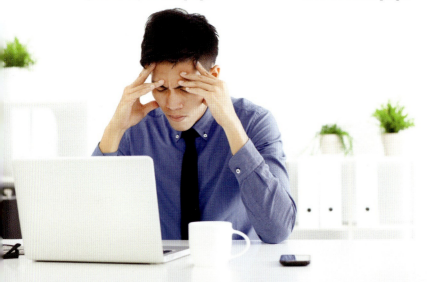

73_Is there a relation between physical exercise and the effect of SiO₂ in the human body?

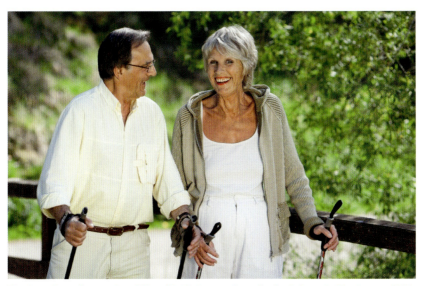

The absorption and processing of silicon is better in case of regular physical exercise than in case of little exercise.

Kudryashova [2000a and b] reports that the intake and processing of silicon in case of regular physical exercise is better than in case of little exercise.

It is recommended to take care of a sufficient individual physical activity, while taking SiO₂.

In this context, the results of Nasolodin et al. [1987] are interesting and have to be mentioned.

These authors examined highly trained top athletes with regard to the consumption of silicon and zinc in the tissue under hard training circumstances. They found out that the consumption of silicon is higher by 30-35 mg/day and that of zinc by 20-25 mg/day than those of normal athletes.

Athletes should take SiO₂ sufficiently by eating food containing silicon or in form of colloidal preparations, better in form of natural zeolite, to maintain their performance level.

74_Can natural zeolite protect hobby athletes and competitive athletes against overload and injuries?

Yes, as oxidative stress, which can be very high in case of competitive athletes, is eliminated. Furthermore, natural zeolite accelerates the regeneration and reduction of injuries. The silicate keeps the sinews, ligaments and muscles elastic. Hobby athletes and competitive athletes from different countries report about performance-enhancing and quick (short-term) regeneration after intake of natural zeolite. The athletes obtained, depending on the type of sport and based on the data from training, natural zeolite in individual doses. Also the duration of intake, that took place during the training or during and after a competition, was applied individually, according to the respective requirements.

Observations of competitive athletes carried out by C. Bandtke and D. Lazik (rowing), who had obtained natural zeolite for a long time, show that this natural remedy can have positive effects on the regeneration process.

75_Are there any studies and sports medical experiences?

In general, there is a controversial discussion about lactate because it can cause a lactate acidosis in cases of an increased physical exercise [Meyer et al. 2004]. The lactate concentration should always be kept low, since lactate acidosis (acidification) can have very harmful effects for the functions of the human organism. The determination of the lactate level is commonly used for the assessment of the training state and health state of the athlete. Dr. Knappitsch and Mag. Schmölzer were able to show with the help of the following examinations on the basis of lactate determination in the blood that by means of administering clinoptilolite-zeolite (PMA zeolite) the lactate level in the blood of athletes could be kept low. [2004 The effect of Panaceo Sport on the lactate levels during physical exercise in humans with the help of a randomised, placebo controlled double-blind study].

They gave men and women who had already done competitive sport for a long time 3 x 3 capsules every day to the meals or 12 capsules before the performance tests for 2 weeks. After 7 and 14 days, a lactate test was carried out on the treadmill. Thanks to the application of clinoptilolite-zeolite, the lactate concentration in the blood could be kept low. They found out that the reduction of the lactate level to below 2 mmol/l led to an enhanced performance by 14 % on an average, below 3 mmol/l to an enhanced performance by 10.2 % and below 4 mmol/l to an enhanced performance by 9.4 %.

Prof. Bachl (University of Vienna, Member of the Medical Commission of the IOC, EOC and ÖOC) assessed this randomised placebo controlled double-blind study as follows:

"To sum up the results from the study, one can say that, in general, all examined active agents, without exception, have the capability to influence different parameters of the endurance performance in a positive way or even to reduce the internal load drastically in case of certain load intensities, which is very important."

76_Could you explain why competitive athletes are satisfied with the intake of natural zeolite?

1. It has been proved scientifically that competitions and excessive training in case of competitive athletes lead to overproduction of free oxygen radicals and lactic acid (oxidative stress).

   Examinations show that free radicals can rise by 6-8 times on an average in case of competitive athletes. If the athletes work out till exhaustion, the production of free radicals can rise twentyfold.

   Natural zeolite can reduce the formation of free radicals and lactate acid and thus accelerate the regeneration process.

2. A shortage of minerals caused by sweating can also lead to regulation problems e.g. with regard to the electrolyte metabolism or acid-base metabolism, and even power loss. For this reason, a sufficient supply of minerals is necessary for the health of competitive athletes but also hobby athletes.

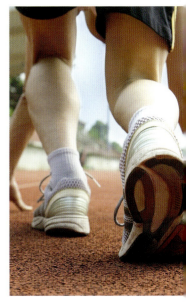

Natural zeolite can meet the mineral need of top athletes selectively by means of selective ion exchange. It is a known fact that the risk of getting injuries rises as a result of excess free radicals and a shortage of minerals in case of competitive athletes. From my point of view, the risk of getting injuries, as it has been the case recently with the soccer players of FC Bayern, can be reduced by applying natural zeolite.

The Austrian record champion SK Rapid Wien has applied PMA zeolite after a long test phase of the medical department already since October 2013 very successfully.

77_Is natural zeolite a doping substance?

No, definitely not. Natural zeolite and the containing SiO_2 offer a physiological protection against pathological overload and injuries. The performance can be provided despite missing minerals. Natural zeolite does not have a toxic effect. It is important that athletes who use natural zeolite during the training and competition drink much water.

78_What are the criteria for the effect of SiO_2 in the connective tissue of the body?

- brain: improvement of the brain metabolism and the mental performance
- mouth: healthy oral mucosa and tongue supplied with blood, good teeth
- immune system: low susceptibility to infections
- hair: much hair, gloss, colour (not grey when old)
- skin: smooth, supplied with blood, firm, elastic
- finger nails: firm, smooth
- cardiovascular system: elastic vessels, normal ECG, good blood and lymph flow
- stomach: tolerance of food, no heartburn
- intestines: normal digestion, normal stool, no or low formation of gases, regular bowel movement
- breathing: strong and deep, no bad breath
- bones: stable, not brittle when old
- sinews/ligaments: strong, elastic
- joints: good formation of cartilage
- muscles: firm, strong

79_What are the consequences of shortage of silicon?

Based on animal experiments and clinical observations, a shortage of silicon can cause diseases involving all organs. According to the present literature, each functional system of the human being can be affected. The following list shows some chosen examples that are meant to provide a picture of the deficiency symptoms. Degeneration due to shortage of silicon has been described for years:

• Many authors report about an accelerated biological ageing process caused by a shortage of silicon.

• Lack of silicon in the body leads to degeneration processes with regard to the joint cartilage. A shortage of silicon can cause arteriosclerosis.

• The chondrocytes that constantly renew the collagenous connective tissue of the joint cartilage are reduced.

• Furthermore, a disturbed silicon metabolism very often results in brittle finger nails and loss of hair.

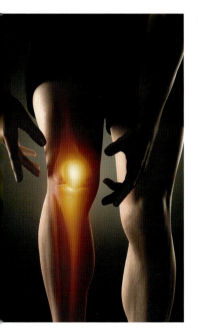

Shortage of silicon causes

• Disturbed calcium and magnesium metabolism in the bones (osteoporosis). Without the presence of silicon there is no regular calcium and magnesium metabolism.

• Arteriosclerosis

• As for arteriosclerosis, there are documented cases where examination results revealed that patients had very low concentrations of silicon in the blood. This means that the cause of arteriosclerosis is related to a disturbed calcium metabolism due to a shortage of silicon.

• Cancer diseases: A number of scientists report about the correlations between shortage of silicon and cancer diseases, which are based on various results from animal experiments and different case studies.

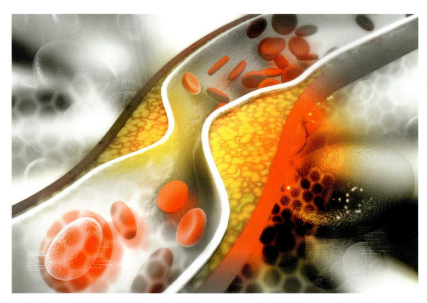

Shortage of silicon causes, among other things, arteriosclerosis and osteoporosis (see picture p. 79).

Furthermore, Voronkov et. al [1975] describe the encapsulation of cancer tumours with calcifications in case of a higher concentration of SiO_2 in the tumour area (animal experiments) as well as an increased amount of silicon in the urine.

- Voronkov et al. [1975] proved loss of hair in case of a shortage of silicon with animal experiments.
- Dermatoses, acne and other skin diseases due to shortage of silicon were observed by many people.
- What is more, a few Russian scientists mention shortage of silicon as a possible cause of diabetes mellitus.
- A shortage of silicon causes senile dementia [Gillette-Guyonnet et al. 2005]

80_Is it true that drinking water containing silicon can prevent Alzheimer's disease?

Yes, it is, results from the EPIDOS study [Gillette-Guyonnet et al. 2005] prove that. This French research group around Sophie Gillette-Guyonnet from the gerontological clinic of the Casselardit hospital Toulouse [2005] assessed the data of a large-scale French long-term study with altogether more than 7,500 female participants aged 75 years and older. The main focus was the relationship between the supply of silicic acid (SiO_2) from drinking water and mental performance.

They found a strong correlation between a reduced mental function at the beginning of the examination and a low silicic acid level of the drinking water. Women with a reduced mental performance had taken approximately 10 %, which is statistically proven, less silicic acid than women with a good mental function. This correlation remained unchanged during the whole duration of observation.

In addition, a sub-group of 383 female participants was examined with regard to the frequency of Alzheimer's disease during the duration of the observation of up to 7 years. According to that, women who took less silicic acid at the beginning of the study had a higher rate of getting dementia than women with a high silicic acid intake.

The researchers concluded that a high silicic acid concentration in the drinking water can provide protection against the loss of mental functions at an advanced age and can even reduce the risk of getting dementia. As a consequence, a shortage of silicon causes senile dementia, not aluminium.

81_Can natural zeolite also have an effect on Alzheimer's disease?

There are research results from animal experiments on rat brains where oxidative stress led to the typical Alzheimer's changes in the brain. When natural zeolite was applied before the application the changes in the brain have not been seen.

Even though relevant studies are missing, one can conclude, in my opinion, from the study results with drinking water that is rich in silicon, the silicates indeed have the power to prevent Alzheimer's disease, considering that they are capable of stopping the biological ageing process. That is, what I have seen when natural zeolite and montmorillonite was taken on a regular basis.

82_Can natural zeolite prevent from osteoporosis?

Prof. Dr. R. Jugdaohsingh emphasises the significance of silicon for the health of bones in a fundamental review. Health of bones means a high density in bone mineral (BMD), which is measurable, and no osteoporosis. He refers to some research results and results of relevant literature.

The basis of a review study of Jugdaohsingh was the increasing number of osteoporosis (reduction of the bone mass) cases and its serious consequences. Among other things, he mentions that 200,000 people suffering from all kinds of bone fractions only in Great Britain every year as a result of osteoporosis. The fractions lead to costs of more than one billion British Pounds. So, while looking for the potential causes of osteoporosis, medical science was also confronted with the shortage of silicon.

The scientific works of Edith Carlisle and Schwarz and Milner are relevant, since they were able to show in animal experiments that silicic acid is inevitable for the normal growth of highly developed animals, including human beings, and that it plays a major role in the formation of connective tissue, especially of bone tissue. A shortage of silicon blocks this type of development.

Numerous cell and tissue culture studies show that zeolite, a natural rock, rich in SiO_2, can stimulate the multiplication of osteoblasts and osteocalcin synthesis of the human being.

Osteoblasts are cells that form bones. Osteocalcin is a special protein that forms bones and that is formed in osteoblasts, and supports the formation of bones.

83_Silicon instead of calcium in therapy and prevention of osteoporosis?

Several research groups have come to this conclusion. In fact, they found out that the presence of silicic acid can help bone fractions heal faster than with calcium applications. The intake of calcium or the consumption of food containing calcium, on the other hand, do not lead to bone health. This is only possible with silicic acid or silicates. Silicic acid can ensure bone health without the application of vitamin D.

84_As you have already mentioned, there are artificial, i.e. synthetic zeolites. How are they produced?

Principally, only aluminium hydroxides and silicon hydroxides are used for the synthesis of artificial zeolites. Both substances are mixed and created in a sodium lye at temperatures between 50° and 90° to form zeolite crystals. The first synthesis of artificial zeolites was carried out by Robert Milton at Linde Air Products Division of Unio Carbide (USA) in the year 1950. The zeolites were called zeolite A and zeolite X.

85_Why is technology interested in zeolites?

The functional characteristics of zeolites found in natural zeolites:
- selective ion exchange
- adsorption (binding)
- molecular sieving function
- catalyst function and
- dehydrations (dryer)

paved the way for the production of artificial zeolites after having adapted the zeolite structures to technical sciences. The technical sciences found advantages in the construction of artificial zeolites in contrast to natural zeolites.

The advantages are:
1. Purity (Natural zeolites contain different substances by nature).
2. The size of the pores and the inner parts of zeolite crystals can be determined and constructed with respect to specific technical reasons, where selective ion exchange plays a role.
3. The fast production for specific reasons is more advantageous for technology than the search for "adequate" nature zeolites.

86_Why are zeolites significant for technology?

Prof. Dr. Hermann Gies and Dr. Bernd Marler begin their article "Zeolite find their way into everyday life. The game with the structures" with the words: "Do you know what 'zeolites' are? No? These fascinating substances are nearly part of our everyday life: no drop of petrol could be produced without them, in detergents they are responsible for 'soft' water, in windows they prevent fogging, and they soak up the humidity in cat litter. Zeolites are very adaptable and offer unlimited fields of application, during the production of fine chemicals, waste water treatment or to divide air into nitrogen and oxygen; they are a great heat accumulator and, above all, environmentally friendly."

87_Could synthetically produced zeolites be significant for health benefits and the medical field?

I have experience with natural zeolites now over close to 25 years in the medical, therapeutic and preventive field, which allows the conclusion that only zeolite, found in nature, should be used for medical reasons, as it corresponds to the nature of human beings. Some functions, disturbing technology, are the ones, perfectly adapted to the nature of human beings and are therefore useful for us. The introduction of artificial zeolites is a new and useful achievement of science and technology. Nature served as a model here. A major advantage of zeolites is, and this should be highlighted, the fact that they are non-toxic, but environmentally friendly. Many sources even characterise zeolites as the basic material of the 21st century.

88_You have characterised natural zeolite and montmorillonite as health-promoting silicates. Which one is better?

Both silicates have their specific functional characteristics. My experiences show, that applying both silicates as a mixture, combining both functional characteristics, will give the best results for health.

89_Could you describe what is specific about montmorillonites?

From my point of view, I would always use montmorillonite instead of bentonite. Bentonite has a percentage of less than 50 % montmorillonite. Montmorillonite is "bentonite" with a percentage of more than 50 % montmorillonite. Montmorillonite has the functional characteristic of ion exchange and adsorption. As montmorillonite is a layered clay originating from weathered tuff, this processes of action are different from those of natural zeolite, however, with the same aim.

90_Main characteristics of montmorillonites that are important for human beings because of their regulative and healing effect

- **Selective ion exchange:** the selective ion exchange takes place via the cations deposited in the spaces within the layered silicate. These can, when the montmorillonite enters the intestines, replace the toxic substances there. NH_4 (ammonia), lead (Pb), caesium (Cs), strontium (Sr), mercury (Hg) and other toxic substances that can be found in the human body, have a great affinity (attraction) to the layers of the silicate and are attracted, absorbed and bound (adsorption). In the released receptors of the body the cations such as magnesium (Mg), potassium (K), sodium (Na), iron (Fe), zinc (Zn) etc. can be absorbed and fulfil their function.
- **Adsorption:** with the help of adsorption, the montmorillonite is capable of binding and neutralising toxic substances that have been removed from the cells and the connective tissue. Adsorption derives from the Latin verb adsorbere, which means to bind. The macropores and micropores of montmorillonite have a huge surface. 1 gramme of montmorillonite can develop a surface of 700-800 m^2 and thus bind and neutralise huge amounts of toxic substances and toxic substances in the human body.

Usually, adsorption and ion exchange are functionally coupled in montmorillonite and natural zeolite. Montmorillonite, however, can not only bind the harmful and toxic substances that were removed from the connective tissue and cells via ion exchange, but also those that can be found in the intestines. This also applies to certain bacteria, fungi and viruses.

91_Which healing effect and other effects does the montmorillonite have?

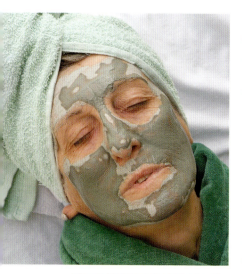

Montmorillonite used as a facial mask.

Montmorillonite has already been applied for centuries in human medicine and veterinary medicine, among other things:

- as a pharmaceutical helping agent
- for the detoxification and removal of toxic substances
- to remove and bind radionuclides (radioprotection)
- for the treatment of chronic diseases as internal and external use
- for the treatment of skin diseases (internal and external use)
- for the treatment of pain (external use)
- for beauty treatments (facial masks)
- for the treatment of disorders of the digestive system, especially in case of diarrhoea

The effects of montmorillonite have been proved:
- healing of wounds
- removal of toxic substances and radionuclides
- relief in case of insect bites
- relief in case of irritable stomach disorders
- immediate relief in case of diarrhoea
- support during intestinal care e.g. medical drug therapy and chemotherapy
- intestinal cleansing

92_What is the detox effect of montmorillonite?

In the past centuries, montmorillonite has been widely applied because of its detoxifying effect with regard to toxins, toxic substances and radionuclides in the human body and animal body. Why?

Montmorillonite binds the following substances in the human and animal body:

- insecticides
- herbicides
- chlorinated carbonates
- ethanol
- methanol

- bacterial endotoxins
- biogenous amins
- heavy metals
- ammonia

[Allison et al. 1974; Carringer et al. 1975]

93_Does montmorillonite remove radionuclides?

In case of cattle and sheep, the radioisotope caesium 134 could be reduced drastically by adding 10 % montmorillonite via adsorption and ion exchange of montmorillonite [Schwarz et al. 1989].

The administration of montmorillonite as an additional food for agricultural livestock can prevent radioactively contaminated food (animal products, meat and milk) and thus harm to the health of human beings.

After the nuclear disaster in Chernobyl montmorillonite and natural zeolite were effectively applied for the removal of radionuclides (caesium 137 and strontium 90). This combination with vitamins and the alga spirulina turned out to be particularly effective [Bgatova and Novoselov 2000]. Equipment, cars and house walls contaminated with radionuclides were treated with montmorillonite alkaline solutions.

94_What are the characteristics of montmorillonites?

Protection of the mucous membranes of the digestive system

With peroral (via the mouth) administration the mucous membrane of the stomach and intestines obtains a thin protective film made of montmorillonite gel with the result that the effect of noxious agents (pathogenic factors) is reduced and the nerve endings of the stomach and the intestines are pacified.

This way the effect of acids, which can cause inflammations in the intestines, is reduced. Numerous scientists explain this mucous membrane protection with a modification caused by montmorillonite of the glycoprotein synthesis of the mucous membrane of the stomach and the intestines. This is a singular protective effect in the intestines.

95_What does montmorillonite do against pathogenic bacteria?

The prophylactic effect of montmorillonite with regard to infections in the gastro-intestinal tract is known. There are some models of explanation:

- binding of pathogenic bacteria (that make sick) to the montmorillonite
- influence of montmorillonite on the population dynamics of bacteria

It has been proved that montmorillonite can selectively influence different bacterial populations. The pH level and nutrition disposition of the bacteria play a decisive role [Schwarz et al. 1989]. **Preventive intake of montmorillonite protects against infections.**

96_Does montmorillonite also have an anti-viral effect?

The binding of viruses with the help of montmorillonite has been proved in numerous studies [Schwarz et al. 1989]. It has to be kept in mind, however, that the virus binding capacity of montmorillonite cannot be compared with pathogenic inactivation. It is possible to reduce or prevent the pathogenic effect of enterocytes by means of adsorption and the virus binding capacity of montmorillonite. **A regular intake of montmorillonite will protect against influenza.**

97_Does montmorillonite have an anti-fungal effect?

With the help of montmorillonite a strong effect on the fungal mycelia in the intestines was proved. The widespread human-pathogenic fungus "histomona capsulatum" is blocked with the help of montmorillonite [Lavie and Stotzky 1986].

Electro-microscopically, a montmorillonite film that embraces the mycelium (fungal net) was found. As a consequence, the gas adsorption, nutrition as well as the metabolism product release of the fungal mycelium was reduced. **As a result, montmorillonite can be seen a good help in case of fungal diseases.**

98_Montmorillonite is characterised as a pharmaceutical supply agent. What does that mean?

The shown physicochemical characteristics: ion exchange, adsorption, swelling capacity and thixotropy of montmorillonite have provided sufficient reasons to use montmorillonite as a pharmaceutical supply agent. To put it into other words, with the help of montmorillonite effects of medical drugs can be weakened or enforced or even adapted to a certain purpose. Similar observations could be made with regard to natural zeolite.

99_Special bed clothes from quartz yarn? Is that possible at all?

In fact, there are special bed clothes from quartz yarn (SiO_2) that are called organic ceramic bed ware.

Some time ago I received scientific information material from the director of the company for natural beds "Samina" in Frastanz (Austria), Dr. hc. Dipl. Psych. Günter W. Amann-Jennson. There is a great variety of bed ware from organic ceramic, among other things, bed toppers, bed duvets, pillows, bed clothes etc.

This range of specific organic ceramic bed ware consists of 60 % cotton tissue or spun sheep's wool and of 40 % organic ceramic yarn that is also called quartz yarn or SiO_2 silicon dioxide yarn.

The special SiO_2 yarn is produced as follows. First of all, quartz (i.e. pure SiO_2) is melted to a quartz liquid at a temperature of 1,600° C. This melted quartz liquid serves as a basis for the next step where very fine yarn is produced by means of a special procedure. This yarn, which consists of crystalline SiO_2 molecules, inherits all characteristics of silicic acid, which have already been described. For example, the yarn has piezo-electrical and pyro-(warmth) electrical characteristics.

In practice, the special SiO_2 yarn is activated by human energy radiation (in form of warmth), which is similar to the battery in a quartz watch. The energy that the human skin provides in form of warmth has frequencies of 8-10 nanometres wavelength. These reflect the infra-red area. They stimulate frequencies in the SiO_2 molecule, which leads to bio-resonance and the soporific effect.

The ceramic bed ware

- supports relaxation and de-stressing as well as the sleeping process,
- improves microcirculation,
- improves the transport of oxygen and nutrients to the cells,
- promotes regeneration and healing (pain-relieving, anti-inflammatory),
- increases the activity of leucocytes and strengthens defence,
- stimulates the lymphatic system and improves detoxification of the tissue,
- improves the elimination of fats, chemicals and toxins from the blood, leading to reduction of the acidic level and rejuvenating/regenerating effect on the nervous system.

My wife and I use organic ceramic bed duvets and are both satisfied with the result, i.e. a good sleep. In this context, I would like to mention that we have published results in a previous work [Hecht and Hecht-Savoley 2008] that prove the soporific effect of clinoptilolite-zeolite powder intake on the basis of measurements with an ambulant automatic electrophysiological sleep analyser.

100_There are earth-eating peoples that are called geophageous peoples. Are they endangered? Earths are aluminium silicates?

There are studies and experiences that prove that geophageous peoples are very healthy. As an example I would like to mention a report of Alexander von Humboldt [Alexander von Humboldt's views of nature, 1st volume, Stuttgart, Cotta, 1859, page 163]:

"Along the coasts of Cumana, New Barcelona, and Caracas, which are visited by the Franciscan monks of Guyana as they return from their missions, the legend of the people on the Orinoco who eat earth is widespread. On our return trip from the Rio Negro (on June 6, 1800), after we had navigated down the Orinoco for 36 days, we spent a day at the mission where the earth-eating Otomacs reside. The earth that the Otomacs eat is a mild, oily loam, a true potter's clay of a yellow-grey hue, coloured with a bit of iron oxide. They choose it carefully, seeking it in certain banks on the edge of the Orinoco and the Meta. They differentiate the taste of different types of earth, and not all loams appeal equally to their taste. They knead this earth into balls of 4 to 6 inches diameter and burn the outside with a weak flame until the crust turns reddish. The ball is moistened again before it is eaten. These Indians are for the most part wild people who abhor cultivating plants.

The Franciscan monk who lives among them as a missionary assures us that he has noticed no change in the health of the Otomacs during the times when they eat this earth. The simple facts then are these: The Indians consume great quantities of loam with no harm to their health; they themselves consider the loam to be foodstuff – that is, upon eating it, they feel full for a long while [...]."

In the book of Dr. W. Price [1997] with the title: "Diet and physical degeneration" you can read the following, among other things. Examinations on geophageous peoples in the Ands, central Africa and the Aborigines in Australia showed that the inhabitants eat clay balls, dipped in water. The explanation of the people was that they wanted to prevent a "bad stomach".

Another interesting remark: SiO_2 and clay are said to have played a role in the origin of life on earth. The Bible says: "And the Lord God formed man of the clay* of the ground, and breathed into his nostrils the breath of life; and man became a living soul." [1. Moses Genesis 2.7 Old Testament]

*: Some bibles use the word loam or dust

Many scientists represent and have proved, based on experiments, the role of clay minerals containing silicon in the origin of life on earth.

Adam was also called "earthling" [Pohl 2008]. When humans have originated from earth, why should earth, consisting of aluminium silicates, be unhealthy? I can answer the question on the basis of my experiences with the daily intake of natural zeolite and mont-morillonite for 15 years with a clear "Yes".

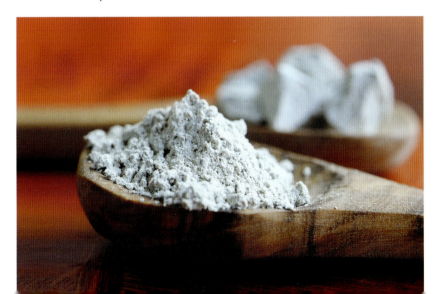

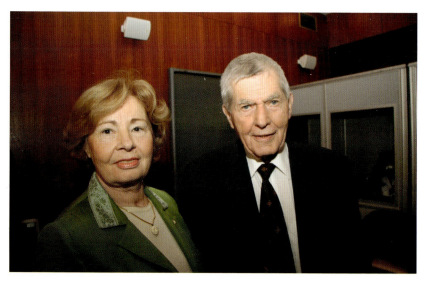

Natural zeolite expert meeting 2011 in Villach/Austria: Dr. med. Ilse Triebnig (Villach) and Prof. Dr. med. habil. Karl Hecht (Berlin) talking.

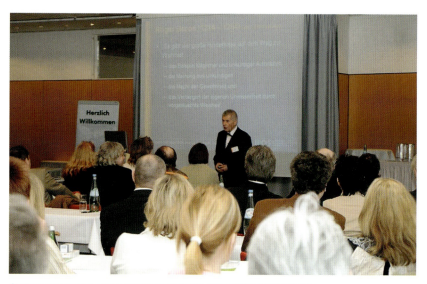

Conference of the International Academy Oxidative Stress IFOS 2008 in Berlin.
Prof. Dr. Karl Hecht during his presentation on the maintenance of health with natural zeolite in a polluted environment in front of 200 participants.

Literature

Allison, D. G.; R. W. Dougherty; E. F. Bucklin; E. E. Snyder (1974): Grain overload in cattle and sheep. Chance in microbial populatios. Amerik. J. Vet. Res. 36, p. 181

Bauer, J. (1994): Die Alzheimer-Krankheit. Neurobiologie, Psychosomatik, diagnostik und Therapie. Schattenauer Verlag, Stuttgart, New York

BfR (2005): Keine Alzheimer-Gefahr durch Aluminium aus Bedarfsgegenständen. Aktualisierte gesundheitliche Bewertung Nr. 033/2007 des BfR (Bundesministerium für Risikobewertung) vom 13. Dezember 2005

Bgatova, N. P.; Ya. B. Novoselov (2000): Anwendung der biologisch-aktiven Nahrungsergänzungsmittel in Form von Naturmineralien zur Detoxikation des Organismus. (russian) Ekor, Novosibirsk, p. 1-238 Ispolzovanie biologičeski aktivnykh pitsherykh dobavok na osnove prirodnykh mineralov ra detoksikazii organisma.

Blagitko, E. M.; I. A. Volkova (1999): Litovit als Komponente einer komplexen Therapie bei obliterarender Arteriosklerose der Gefäße der unteren Extremitäten. Abstraktband: Materialien der wissenschaftlich-praktischen Konferenz „Naturmineralien im Dienste des Menschen: Mineralien, Umwelt und Leben". Ekor-Verlag, Novosibirsk, p. 93-94 (russian) Litovit v Kačestve komponenta Kompleksnogo lečeniya pri obliteriruyntshem ateroskleroze sosudov nishnikh Konečnostey v. Materialny naučno-praktičeskoy. Konferenzii s meshdunarodnym učastem: Prirodnye mineraly na slushbe čeloveka. Mineralnaya sreda i shizn. Ekor, Novosibirsk

Blagitko, E. M.; F. T. Yashina (2000): Prophylaktische und therapeutische Eigenschaften des Naturzeoliths. Ekor, Novosibirsk, p. 1-158 (russian) Profilaktičeskie i lečebnye svoystva prirodykh zeolitov. Febral, Novosibirsk, ISBN 5-85618-115-8

Bundesverband der Lebensmittelchemiker(-innen) im öffentlichen Dienst (BLG) (2013): Aluminium in Lebensmitteln. www.lebensmittel.org

Candy, J. M.; J. Klinowski; R. H. Perry; E. K. Perry; A. Fairbairn; A. E. Oakley; T. A. Carpenter; J. R. Atack; G. Blessed; J. A. Edwardson (1986):
Aluminosilicates and senile plaque formation in Alzheimer's desease. Lancet, p. 354-357

Candy, J. M.; F. K. McArthur; A. E. Oakley; G. A. Taylor; CP.L. H. Chen; S. A. Mountfort; I. E. Thompson; P. R. Chalker; H. E. Pishop; K. Beyreuther; G. Perry; M. K. Ward; C. N. Martyn; J. A. Edwardson (1992): Aluminium accumilation in relation to senile plaque and neurofibrillary tangle formation in the brains of patients with renal failure. J. Neurol. Sci 107, p. 210-218

Carlisle, E. M. (1986a): Silicon in Animal Tissues and Fluids. Academic Press. Inc. New York

Carlisle, E. M. (1986b): Silicon as an essential trace element in animal nutrition. In: Ciba Foundation Symp. 121: Silicon biochemistry., John Wiley u. Sons, Chichester u. a, p. 123-139

Carlisle, E. M. (1986c): Silicon. In: W. Mertz (ed): Trace Elements in Human and Animal Nutrition. 5th edn. Academic Press, Orlando, Florida

Carlisle, E. M. (1986d): Effect of dietary silicon and aluminium on silicon and aluminium levels in rat brain. Alzheimer Dis. Assoc. Dis 1

Carringer, R. D.; B. J. Weber; T. J. Monaco (1975): Adsorption-Desorption of selected pesticides by organic matter and montmorillonit. J. Agri. Food Chem. 23

Chafi, A. H.; J. J. Hauw; G. Rancurel; J. P. Berry; C. Galle (1991): Absence of aluminium in Alzheimer's disease brain tissue: electron microprobe and ion microprobe studies. Neurosci Lett 123, p. 61-64

Čuikova und Voshakov (1999): Anwendung von Natur-Klinoptilolith-Zeolith (Litovito) bei akuter Virushepatitis an Menschen. Forschungsbericht des Lehrstuhls für Infektionskrankheiten der staatlichen Universität Tomsk (russian)

Daskaloff,. N. (2005): froximun: Verhalten von isotopenmarkiertem aktiviertem Klinoptilolith-Zeolith während des Durchgangs im Verdauungstrakt. Auszüge vorliegender Forschungsergebnisse, November 2006, p. 41-42

Deitsch, R. J. (2005): Natural Cellular Defence. Scientific Research Monograph

Duffus, J. H. (2001): Definitons of heavy metal: Survey

of current usage. http://www.iupac.org/publications/ ci/2001/november/heavymetals_tl.html

EFSA (European Food Safety Authority) (2008): Technical Report: Dietary exposure to aluminium-containing food additives. Scientific Opinion of the Panel on Food Additives, Flavourings, Processing Aids and Food Contact Materials on a request from European Commission on Safety of Aluminium from dietary intake. The EFSA Journal 754, p. 1-4

EFSA (European Food Safety Authority) (2013): Technical Report: Epster, Publikation EN 411., Parma, Italy

Gillette-Guyonnet, S.; S. Andrieu; F. Nourhashemi; V. de La Guèronnière; H. Grandjean; B. Vellas (2005): Cognitive impairment and composition of drinking water in women: findings of EPIDOS Study. Service de Médecine interne et Gérontologie Clinique, Hôpital Casselardit, Touluse, France. Am J Clin Nutr 81, p. 897-902

Goldstein, F. (1932): In: K. Kaufmann (1997): Silizium, Heilung durch Ursubstanz. Helfer Verlag, E. Schwabe GmbH, Bad Homburg

Good, P. F.; D. P. Perl; L. M. Bierer; J. Schmeidler (1992): Selective accumulation of aluminum and iron in the neurofibrillary tangles of Alzheimer's disease: a laser microprobe (LAMMA) study. Ann Neurol 31, p. 286-292

Hecht, K.; E. N. Hecht-Savoley (2005, 2008): Naturmineralien, Regulation, Gesundheit. Schibri-Verlag, Berlin, Milow, 1. and 2. edition, ISBN 3-937895-05-1

Hecht, K.; E. Hecht-Savoley (2008): Klinoptilolith-Zeolith – Siliziummineralien und Gesundheit. Spurbuchverlag, Baunach; 2. edition 2010, 3. edition 2011, ISBN 987-3-88778-322-8

von Humboldt, A. (1859): Ansichten der Natur. 1. vol., Stuttgart Cotta p.. 163-98

Ivković, S. (2006): Tumorkrankheiten. Wissenschaftlicher Vortrag (Manuskript) zur Megamin Produktvorstellung

Kudryashova, N. I. (2000a): Gesund durch Silizium. Moskwa, Obraz-Kompanidat (russian) Kremnewoje sdorowje

Kudryashova, I. (2000b): Behandlung mit Ton. (russian) Moskau Opraz Kompanisdat., p. 1-94

Landsberg, J. P.; B. McDonald; F. Watt (1992): Absence of aluminium in neuritic plaque cores in Alzheimer's disease. Nature 360, p. 65-68

Lang, U. (2012): Terra sigillata – Zur Geschichte antiker Heilerden. Deutsches Ärzteblatt 109/41, p. C1627-C1628

Lavie, S.; G. Stotzky (1986): Adhesion of the clay minerals montmorillonite, kaolinite and attapulgite reduces respiration of histoplasma capsulatum. Appl. Environm. Microbiol. 51, 1, p. 65-73

Lelas, T.; V. Lelas (2004): Präliminere Studie über die Verwendung von Megamin zur Senkung der Anteile von Lactaten und Ammonium im menschlichen Körper. Wissenschaftlicher Bericht, Zagreb

Malsy, A.; D. Döbelin (2004): Beilagen für den Geographie-Unterricht. Institut für Geologie, Univeristät Bern

Martyn, C. N.; C. Osmond; J. A. Edwardson; D. J. P. Barker; E. C. Harris; R. F. Lacey (1989): Geographical relation between Alzheimer's desease and aluminiuum in drinking water. Lancet 8, p. 59-62

Meyer, T.; O. Faude; J. Scharhag; A. Urbausen; W. Kindermann (2004): Is lactic acidosis a cause of exercise induced hyperventilaion at the respiratory compensation point? Br J Sorts Med 38, p. 622-625

Montinaro, M.; D. Uberti; G. Maccarinelli; S. A. Bonini; G. Ferrari-Toninelli; M. Memo (2013): Dietary zeolite supplementation reduces oxidative damage and plaque generation in the brain of an Alzheimer's disease mouse model. Department of Biomedical Sciences and Biotechnologies, University of Brescia, 25123 Brescia, Italy. Life Sci, http://dx.doi.org/10.1016/j.lfs.2013.03.008

Nasolodin, V. V.; V. Ya Rusin; V. A. Vorobev (1987): Zinc and silicon metabolism in highly trained athletes under hard physical stress (russian). Vaprosy pitaniya 4, p. 37-39

Pavelič, K; M. Hadžija (2003): Medical Applications of Zeolites. In: S. M. Auerbach, K. A. Carrado; P. K. Dutta (eds): Handbook of Zeolite Science and Technology. Marcel Dekker Inc. New York, Basel

Pavelič, K.; S. Schimpf; J. Meyer-Wegner (2004): Zeolithe. Die Kraft aus dem Urgestein der Erde. 1-98, no Verlagsangabe

Pohl, C. (2008): Lehmdoktors Fibel. Edition www.lehm-doktor.de, Books on Demand GmbH, Norderstedt, 144 Seiten, ISBN 978-3-8370-7428- 4

Price, W. A. (1997): Ernährung und körperliche Degeneration.

Rifat, S. L.; M. R. Eastwood; D. R. Crapper McLachlan; P. B. Corey (1990): Effects of exposure of miners to aluminium powder. Lancet 336, p. 1162-1165

Scholl, O.; K. Letters (1959): Über die Kieselsäure und ihre physiologische Wirkung in der Geriatrie. München, Medizinische Wochenschrift 101/5, p. 2321-2325

Schwarz, R. (1989): Der Stand der Forschung zur sogenannten prämorbiden Krebspersönlichkeit. In: R. Verres; M. Hasenbring (Hrsg.): Psychosoziale Onkologie. Jahrbuch der Medizinischen Psychologie, vol. 3, Springer, Berlin

Shakov, Y. I. (1999): In: O. A. Veretenina; N. V. Kostina; T. Novoselova; Y. B. Vovoselov; A. G. Ronnisonn (2003): Litovit. Novosibirsk, p. 38-39 (russian)

Thieme Chemistry (Hrsg.) (2013): Georg Thieme Verlag, Stuttgart

Veretenina, O. A.; N. V. Kostina; T. I. Novoselova; Ja. B. Novoselov; A. G. Roninson (2003): Litovit. Novosibirsk, Izdar (Verlag) Ekor, p. 1-103 (russian), ISBN 5-85618-107-7

Voronkov, M. G.; G. L. Zelchan; E. Lukevitz (1975): Silizium und Leben. Akademie-Verlag, Berlin

Warnke, U.; P. Hensinger (2013): Steigende „Burn out"-Indizien durch technische und elektromagnetische Felder des Mobil- und Kommunikationsfunks. Forschungsbericht. Herausgeber: Kompetenzinitiative zum Schutz von Mensch, Umwelt und Demokratie, Januar

White, K. N.; A. L. Ejim; R. C. Walton; A. P. Brown; R. Jugdaohsingh; J. J. Powell; C. R. McCrohan (2008): Avoidance of aluminum toxicity in freshwater snails involved intracelluar silicon-aluminum biointeraction. Environ Sci Technol 42(6), p. 2189-2894

Yakymenko, I.; E. Sidorek; D. Henshel; S. Kyrylenko (2014): Mikrowellen niedriger Intensität: Ein neues Oxidationsmittel für lebende Zellen. Oxid. Antioxid. Med. Sci. 3, p. 1-3

Ziskoven, R. (1997a): Rationeller Einsatz eines lebenswichtigen Mineralstoffs. In: Magnesium als Therapieprinzip. TW Taschenbuch – Medizin. G. Braun, Karlsruhe, vol. 25, p. 7-20

Ziskoven, R. (1997b): Einsatzgebiet eines natürlichen Basistherapeutikums. In: Magnesium als Therapieprinzip. TW Taschenbuch – Medizin. G. Braun, Karlsruhe, vol. 25, p. 21-32

Bibliographic data

Dr. med. Dr. med. habil. Karl Hecht

Born on 15/02/1924 in Wohlmirstedt

doctor, scientist, university professor, active retiree

1950-1955	studies at the Medical Faculty (Charité) of the Humboldt University Berlin 1957
1957	Dr. med.
1970	habilitation
1971	appointed professor of the Section Neurophysiology at the Academy of Sciences in the German Democratic Republic
1977	appointed professor and founding director at the Institute for experimental and clinical pathophysiology at the Charité of the Humboldt University in Berlin (pathophysiology = science of the functions of the development of diseases)

Main focuses of his research work:
Stress, sleep, chrono, environment, space medicine, blood pressure regulation, mineral metabolism, neuropsychobiology, regulation peptides, health sciences, neuro sciences.

publications:
more than 800 scientific papers in national magazines and international magazines and anthologies; 53 scientific reference books and non-fiction books; 28 patents

support of scientific junior researchers:
accompanied 173 doctoral students.

Elected and honorary memberships (examples):
– Member of the International Academy of the Sciences Health and Ecology, Innsbruck
– Member of the International Academy for Astronautics (Paris)
– Foreign Member of the Russian Academy of Sciences (Moscow)
– Honorary member of the physiological society Cuba, Havanna
– Honorary member of the Czech Medical Society "Purkinje", Prague
– Presidium member of the "World Organization for Scientific Cooperation" (WOSCO)
– Presidium member of the "International Committee GEOCHANGE on Global Geological and Environmental Change"
– Honorary president of the European Academy for Medical Prevention (Berlin)
– Honours: Juri Gagarin medal and Oleg Gazenko medal for space medical contributions